The Science of AIDS

The Science of AIDS

. . .

READINGS FROM
SCIENTIFIC AMERICAN MAGAZINE

W. H. FREEMAN AND COMPANY
New York

Library of Congress Cataloging-in-Publication Data

The Science of AIDS : a Scientific American reader.
    p.   cm.
  Articles originally appeared in the Oct. 1988 issue of
Scientific American.
  Bibliography: p.
  Includes index.
  ISBN 0-7167-2036-1
  1. AIDS (Disease)   I. Scientific American.
RC607.A26S38   1989
616.97'92—dc19   88-32221
                                                   CIP

The ten chapters and the epilogue in this book originally
appeared as articles and the closing essay in the October,
1988 issue of SCIENTIFIC AMERICAN.

Printed in the United States of America

1234567890 RRD 765454321089

CONTENTS

Foreword   vii
Jonathan Piel

1   **The AIDS Epidemic**   1
    Robert C. Gallo and Luc Montagnier

2   **The Molecular Biology of the AIDS Virus**   13
    William A. Haseltine and Flossie Wong-Staal

3   **The Origins of the AIDS Virus**   27
    Max Essex and Phyllis J. Kanki

4   **The Epidemiology of AIDS in the U.S.**   39
    William L. Heyward and James W. Curran

5   **The International Epidemiology of AIDS**   51
    Jonathan M. Mann, James Chin, Peter Piot and Thomas Quinn

6   **HIV Infection: The Clinical Picture**   63
    Robert R. Redfield and Donald S. Burke

7   **HIV Infection: The Cellular Picture**   75
    Jonathan N. Weber and Robin A. Weiss

8   **AIDS Therapies**   85
    Robert Yarchoan, Hiroaki Mitsuya and Samuel Broder

9   **AIDS Vaccines**   101
    Thomas J. Matthews and Dani P. Bolognesi

10 **The Social Dimensions of AIDS**   111
    Harvey V. Fineberg

EPILOGUE
AIDS: An Unknown Distance Still to Go   123
Lewis Thomas

The Authors   125

Bibliographies   127

Index   130

Foreword

Had a novelist sought a plot device that would lay bare the strengths, weaknesses and contradictions in the social fabric, the policy-making institutions and the moral vision of contemporary humanity, he or she could not have hit upon a better one than the AIDS epidemic. A blood-borne pathogen spread by sexual contact, drug abuse and advanced techniques of medical therapy leaps oceans, aided by a network of rapid, convenient air travel. It quietly gains footholds in both the northern and southern hemispheres, in market economies and planned economies. The virus attacks, cripples and destroys the body's only defense against disease: the immune system. Understandably the human immunodeficiency virus (HIV) has provoked intense fear and an angry backlash against public institutions and science itself. Actually their record to date has been one of extraordinary achievement. Within two years of the recognition of AIDS as a disease, the infectious agent had been identified. That work paid a dividend: an antibody test useful in protecting the blood supply and identifying infected individuals. Investigators have now opened several promising lines of chemotherapy and immunotherapy. All of those achievements, described by leading workers in the October, 1988 issue of SCIENTIFIC AMERICAN and reproduced in this volume, have their roots in basic research — research performed with no inkling that such a severe challenge was in the offing. Had the epidemic broken out in the 1960's or early 1970's, neither the way in which it attacks the immune system nor the virus itself could have been understood. It is unlikely that even the most ambitious, tightly focused crash program could have produced the results that emerged from fundamental inquiry into scientific and clinical questions.

The contributors to *The Science of AIDS* are confident that our species can meet this challenge. Yet caution tempers optimism. The therapeutic strategies are promising but the therapies are not yet at hand; HIV is a labile organism — it could become more virulent or evolve into coexistence. The dimensions of the epidemic are not yet clear, but it is certain that the cost in life and in treasure will be high. In the U.S., at least, a coherent institutional mechanism for guiding the efforts to combat AIDS has yet to be devised. HIV has already begun to force reexamination of how we view individual rights and professional ethics; such questions are likely to become even more vexing if the epidemic spreads beyond its primary risk groups. In a social atmosphere of tension, uncertainty and, inevitably, misinformation, *The Science of AIDS* serves thoughtful citizens as an accurate point of reference for logical thinking and constructive response.

Jonathan Piel
Editor, SCIENTIFIC AMERICAN

The Science of AIDS

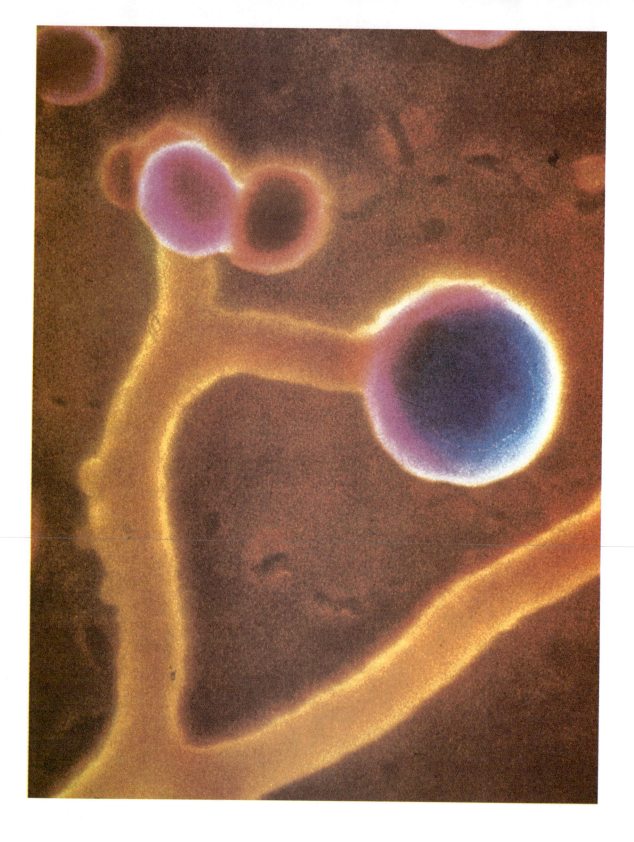

The AIDS Epidemic

*In their first collaborative article the investigators who discovered
HIV recount the discovery and offer prospects for vaccine,
for therapy and for the epidemic.*

. . .

Robert C. Gallo and Luc Montagnier

As recently as a decade ago it was widely believed that infectious disease was no longer much of a threat in the developed world. The remaining challenges to public health there, it was thought, stemmed from noninfectious conditions such as cancer, heart disease and degenerative diseases. That confidence was shattered in the early 1980's by the advent of AIDS. Here was a devastating disease caused by a class of infectious agents—retroviruses—that had first been found in human beings only a few years before. In spite of the startling nature of the epidemic, science responded quickly. In the two years from mid-1982 to mid-1984 the outlines of the epidemic were clarified, a new virus—the human immunodeficiency virus (HIV)—was isolated and shown to cause the

disease, a blood test was formulated and the virus's targets in the body were established.

Following that initial burst, progress has been steady, albeit slower. Yet in some respects the virus has outpaced science. No cure or vaccine is yet available, and the epidemic continues to spread; disease-causing retroviruses will be among the human population for a long time. In view of that prospect, it is essential to ask where we stand in relation to AIDS in 1988. How was HIV discovered and linked to AIDS? How does the virus cause its devastation? What are the chances that AIDS will spread rapidly outside the known high-risk groups? What are the prospects for a vaccine? For therapy? How can the epidemic most effectively be fought? Those are some of the questions this chapter and this SCIENTIFIC AMERICAN Reader have set out to answer.

Like other viruses, retroviruses cannot replicate without taking over the biosynthetic apparatus of a cell and exploiting it for their own ends. What is unique about retroviruses is their capacity to reverse the ordinary flow of genetic information—from DNA to RNA to proteins (which are the cell's structural and functional molecules). The genetic material of a retrovirus is RNA. In addition, the retrovi-

Figure 1 NEW AIDS-VIRUS PARTICLES burst from a thin tube called microvillus extending from the surface of an infected cell in culture. The micrograph has an enlargement of more than 500,000 diameters. (The colors are artificial.) The virus, which is now called the human immunodeficiency virus (HIV), belongs to the category called retroviruses. It was discovered and linked to AIDS by the authors of this chapter. (Micrograph by Lennart Nilsson of the Karolinska Institute in Stockholm.)

rus carries an enzyme called reverse transcriptase, which can use the viral RNA as a template for making DNA. The viral DNA can integrate itself into the genome (the complement of genetic information) of the host. Having made itself at home among the host's genes, the viral DNA remains latent until it is activated to make new virus particles. The latent DNA can also initiate the process that leads to tumor formation.

Retroviruses and their cancer-causing potential are not new to science. At the beginning of this century several investigators identified transmissible agents in animals that were capable of causing leukemias (cancers of blood cells) as well as solid-tissue tumors. In the succeeding decades retroviruses were identified in many animal species. Yet the life cycle of retroviruses remained obscure until 1970, when Howard M. Temin of the University of Wisconsin at Madison and (independently) David Baltimore of the Massachusetts Institute of Technology discovered reverse transcriptase, confirming Temin's hypothesis that the retroviral life cycle includes an intermediate DNA form, which Temin had called the provirus. The details of viral replication quickly fell into place.

In spite of such discoveries, by the mid-1970's no infectious retroviruses had been found in human beings, and many investigators firmly believed no human retrovirus would ever be found. Their skepticism had several grounds. Many excellent scientists had tried and failed to find such a virus. Moreover, most animal retroviruses had been fairly easy to find, because they replicated in large quantities, and the new virus particles were readily observed in the electron microscope; no such phenomenon had been found in human beings. In spite of this skepticism, by 1980 a prolonged team effort led by one of us (Gallo) paid off in the isolation of the first human retrovirus: human *T*-lymphotropic virus type I (HTLV-I).

HTLV-I infects *T* lymphocytes, white blood cells that have a central role in the immune response. The virus causes a rare, highly malignant cancer called adult *T*-cell leukemia (ATL) that is endemic in parts of Japan, Africa and the Caribbean but is spreading to other regions as well. Two years after the discovery of HTLV-I the same group isolated its close relative, HTLV-II. HTLV-II probably causes some cases of a disease called hairy-cell leukemia as well as *T*-cell leukemias and lymphomas of a more chronic type than those linked to HTLV-I. The two

viruses, however, share some crucial features. They are spread by blood, by sexual intercourse and from mother to child. Both cause disease after a long latency, and both infect *T* lymphocytes. When AIDS was first recognized, these properties took on great additional significance.

The first AIDS cases were diagnosed in 1981 among young homosexual men in the U.S. (see Chapter 4, "The Epidemiology of AIDS in the U.S.," by William L. Heyward and James W. Curran). Although the syndrome was puzzling, it soon became clear that all its victims suffered from a depletion of a specific subset of *T* cells—T4 cells—and that as a result they fell prey to pathogens that would easily be controlled by a healthy immune system (see Chapter 6, "HIV Infection: The Clinical Picture," by Robert R. Redfield and Donald S. Burke). A variety of hypotheses were advanced to explain AIDS, including breakdown of the victims' immune systems following repeated exposure to foreign proteins—or even to sperm—during homosexual intercourse. It seemed more plausible, however, to explain a new syndrome by the appearance of a new infectious agent.

To one of us (Gallo) the likeliest agent was a retrovirus. It had already been shown that the AIDS pathogen, like HTLV-I, could be transmitted by sexual intercourse and by blood. Furthermore, Max Essex of the Harvard School of Public Health had shown that a retrovirus of cats called feline leukemia virus (FeLV) could cause either cancer or immune suppression. Since in most species the infectious retroviruses are closely related, it seemed plausible that the same was true in human beings. Hence the initial hypothesis was that the cause of AIDS was a close relative of HTLV-I. That hypothesis, as it turned out, was wrong. Nonetheless, it was fruitful, because it stimulated the search that led to the correct solution.

The retrovirus hypothesis for the origin of AIDS reached the other one of us in France in the following way. Almost as soon as AIDS was first diagnosed, a working group on the syndrome had been formed by a circle of young clinicians and researchers in France. One member of the group, Jacques Leibowitch of the Raymond Poincaré Hospital in Paris, had had some contact with Gallo's team and carried the HTLV hypothesis back to France. The members of the French group wanted to test that hypothesis, and they had the biological materials to do so, because the group included clinicians with patients

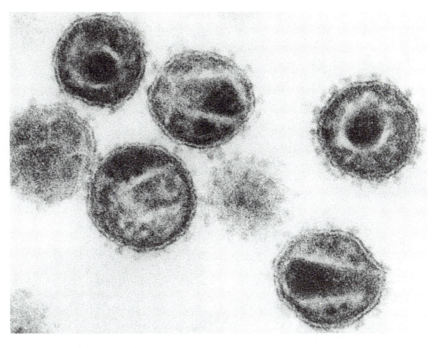

Figure 2 HIV VIRION, or particle, is a sphere 1,000 angstrom units (one ten-thousandth of a millimeter) across. The sphere contains a core that holds the virus's genetic material: RNA. The core is a truncated cone; from the end it appears as a disk. The virion is wrapped in a membrane like that of a cell, from which protein "knobs" extend. The knobs are faintly visible in the micrograph, which has an enlargement of 200,000 diameters. (Micrograph by Hans Gelderblom of the Robert Koch Institute in Berlin.)

afflicted by AIDS or pre-AIDS. What they lacked, however, was the collaboration of virologists experienced in work with retroviruses.

The French author of this article and his colleagues Françoise Barré-Sinoussi and Jean-Claude Chermann at the Pasteur Institute fitted that description. They were engaged in several lines of work on cancer and interferon, including attempts to find retroviruses in patients with cancer, particularly in cultures of lymphocytes. A member of the working group, Willy Rozenbaum of the Salpêtrière Hospital, asked whether they were interested in analyzing tissues from a patient with lymphadenopathy, or swollen glands. (Lymphadenopathy can be an early sign of the process that culminates in AIDS. Such a patient was chosen because finding a virus early in the disease seemed more meaningful than finding one later, when AIDS patients were infected with many opportunistic agents.) The answer was yes, and in January, 1983, a specimen from the swollen lymph node of a young homosexual arrived at Montagnier's laboratory.

The specimen was minced, put into tissue culture and analyzed for reverse transcriptase. After two weeks of culture, reverse-transcriptase activity was detected in the culture medium. A retrovirus was present. But which one? The first possibility that had to be tested was whether the virus was one of the known HTLV's, or perhaps a close relative of them. That possibility was tested using specific HTLV-I reagents supplied by Gallo. The virus did not react significantly with the HTLV-I reagents; a similar result was later obtained with HTLV-II reagents. A strenuous effort was begun to characterize the new agent.

Among the first results of that effort was the finding that the new virus (which was named lymphadenopathy-associated virus, or LAV) grew in T4 cells but not in related cells called T8; that finding was made by David Klatzmann and Jean-Claude Gluckman of the Salpêtrière Hospital in collaboration with the Pasteur group. It was shown that the virus could kill T4 cells or inhibit their growth. Electron micrographs of the new virus were different from those of HTLV-I and resembled those of a retrovirus of horses. A viral protein called P25 (or P24) that is not present in HTLV-I was identified. In collaboration with virologists from the Claude Bernard Hospital a blood test for LAV antibodies was formulated. Several examples of LAV or LAV-like viruses were isolated from homosexual men, hemophiliacs and central Africans.

Early results of applying the blood test were suggestive but not fully conclusive. LAV antibodies were found in a large fraction of lymphadenopathy patients but in only a minority of AIDS patients. Yet the proportion increased as the sensitivity of the test improved. By October, 1983, it had reached 40 percent. At that point one of us (Montagnier) was convinced LAV was the best candidate for the cause of AIDS.

To the other one of us the evidence did not seem so clear. For one thing, results had been obtained (by Gallo and Essex) indicating that some AIDS patients are infected with HTLV-I or a variant of that virus. It is now known that those results stemmed partly from the fact that among people infected with HIV are some who are also infected with the HTLV's. Moreover, only a minority—albeit a substantial one—of AIDS patients had shown serological evidence of LAV infection. In addition, when it was first isolated, LAV could not be grown in large amounts in continuous cell lines. Without large quantities of virus it was difficult to prepare specific LAV reagents that could be used to show that all people with AIDS or pre-AIDS were infected by the same type of virus.

Therefore on the American side much effort was concentrated on growing the pathogen from the blood of AIDS patients in mass, continuous culture. By the end of 1983 that task had been accomplished by the Gallo team: several cell lines had been identified that could support the growth of the new agent (see Figure 7). The first reagents for specifically typing this virus were rapidly made. Employing those reagents, it was shown that 48 isolates obtained beginning in early 1983 from AIDS patients and people in risk groups were all the same type of virus, which was called HTLV-III on the American side. A blood test was formulated and used to show that HTLV-III was present in almost all people with AIDS, in a variable proportion of people at risk of the disease (including people who had received blood contaminated by the virus but had no other risk factors) and in no healthy heterosexuals. The cause of AIDS had been conclusively established.

These results confirmed and extended the ones from France. LAV and HTLV-III were soon shown to be the same virus. Before long an international commission had changed its name to HIV, to eliminate confusion caused by two names for the same entity and to acknowledge that the virus does indeed cause AIDS. Thus contributions from our laboratories—in roughly equal proportions—had demonstrated that the cause of AIDS is a new human retrovirus.

That HIV is the cause of AIDS is by now firmly established. The evidence for causation includes the fact that HIV is a new pathogen, fulfilling the original postulate of "new disease, new agent." In addition, although the original tests found evidence of HIV infection in only a fraction of people with AIDS, newer and more sensitive methods make it possible to find such evidence in almost every individual with AIDS or pre-AIDS. Studies of blood-transfusion recipients indicate that people exposed to HIV who have no other risk factors develop AIDS. The epidemiological evidence shows that in every country studied so far AIDS has appeared only after HIV. What is more, HIV infects and kills the very T4 cells that are depleted in AIDS. Although the causative role of HIV in AIDS has been questioned, to us it seems clear that the cause of AIDS is as well established as that of any other human disease.

Soon after the causation was established, a series of findings began to fill in the scientific picture of HIV. In a remarkably short time the genetic material of the virus was cloned and sequenced (in our laboratories and several others). The genetic complexity of HIV began to emerge when a gene called *tat* was discovered by William A. Haseltine of the Dana-Farber Cancer Institute, Flossie Wong-Staal of the National Cancer Institute and their collaborators (see Chapter 2, "The Molecular Biology of the AIDS Virus," by William A. Haseltine and Flossie Wong-Staal). Such complexity is significant because it underlies the capacity of HIV to remain latent for a long period, then undergo a burst of replication, a

Figure 3 VIRION STRUCTURE is shown in cross section. The knobs consist of a protein called gp120, which is anchored to another protein called gp41. Each knob includes three sets of protein molecules (*box below*). The virus's core includes a protein called p25 or p24. In the core, along with the RNA that carries the virus's genetic information, is an enzyme known as reverse transcriptase. Reverse transcriptase enables the virus to make DNA corresponding to the viral RNA. The DNA inserts itself into the host cell's chromosomes and remains latent until it is activated to make new virus particles.

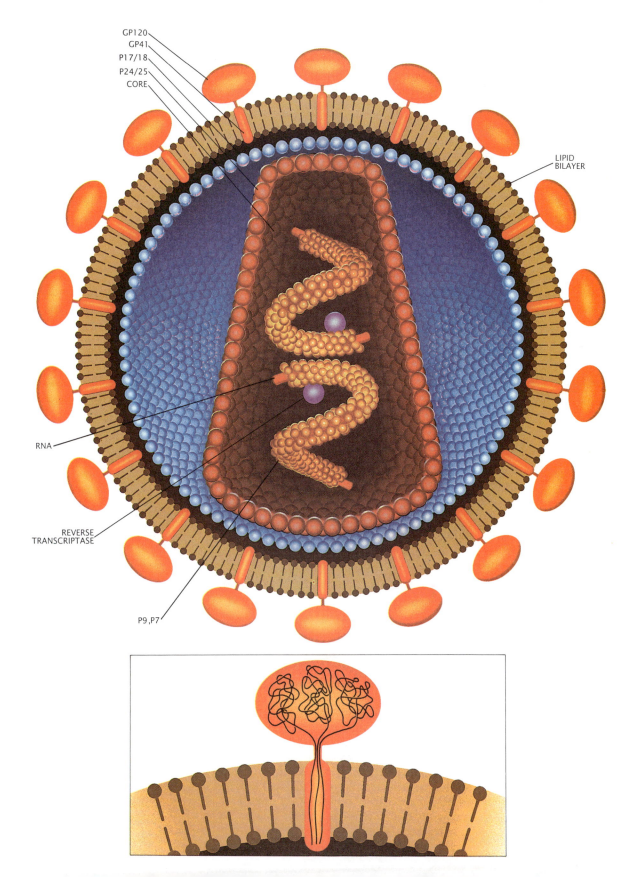

GP120
GP41
P17/18
P24/25
CORE

LIPID
BILAYER

RNA

REVERSE
TRANSCRIPTASE

P9,P7

TYPE OF EVIDENCE	DESCRIPTION
ANIMAL SYSTEMS	Several types of retroviruses can cause severe immune deficiencies in animals. For example, the feline leukemia virus (FeLV) can cause either immune deficiency or cancer, depending on slight genetic variations in the virus. A virus related to HIV, the simian immunodeficiency virus (SIV), can cause AIDS in macaque monkeys. The second AIDS virus, HIV-2, may also cause AIDS in macaques.
EPIDEMIOLOGY	In every country studied so far, AIDS has appeared only after the appearance of HIV. Using the most recent technology, HIV can be isolated from almost 100 percent of the people with AIDS. Earlier in the epidemic, the virus was present in the groups at risk for the disease and in almost no healthy heterosexuals.
BLOOD-TRANSFUSION DATA	A study of people who received blood transfusions in 1982–83 (when the fraction of blood donors infected with HIV was about 1 in 2,000) showed that of 28 people who got AIDS, the virus could be found in all 28. Furthermore, for each recipient who got AIDS an infected donor could be found. Today most of those infected donors have also developed AIDS. Elimination of HIV in blood transfusions by antibody screening has drastically reduced the number of AIDS cases resulting from transfusions.
TEST-TUBE STUDIES	In the laboratory the virus kills the very T4 cells whose depletion is the hallmark of AIDS. It also infects and alters the function of cells of the monocyte-macrophage lineage, which may serve as a reservoir of infection in AIDS patients.

Figure 4 EVIDENCE THAT HIV CAUSES AIDS is by now as firm as that for the causation of any other human disease. As the table shows, the supporting data come from a range of sources, including epidemiology, analysis of blood-serum samples and cell biology.

pattern that may hold the key to the pathology of AIDS.

There were other significant early findings. One of us (Gallo), with his colleagues Mikulas Popovic and Suzanne Gartner, showed that HIV could infect not only the T4 cell but also another type of white blood cell, the macrophage. The same one of us, working with his colleagues Beatrice H. Hahn, George M. Shaw and Wong-Staal, found HIV in brain tissues. It seems possible that the macrophage, which can cross the blood-brain barrier, may bring virus into the brain, explaining the central-nervous-system pathology seen in many AIDS patients.

How the virus infects both T4 cells and macrophages became clear when Robin A. Weiss of the Chester Beatty Laboratories and, independently, Klatzmann and the Pasteur group showed that HIV enters its target cells by interacting with the molecule called CD4 (see Chapter 7, "HIV Infection: The Cellular Picture," by Jonathan N. Weber and Robin A. Weiss). CD4 has a significant role in the immune function of T4 lymphocytes and also serves as a marker for that group of cells. The early work by the British and French teams showed that HIV infects cells by binding to CD4. Hence only cells bearing that marker can be infected. (Although CD4 is the

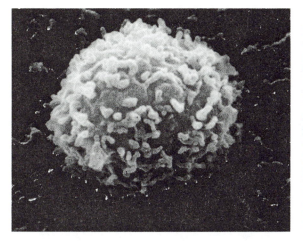

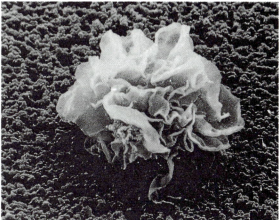

Figure 5 MAIN TARGETS OF HIV are two white blood cells: the lymphocyte and the macrophage. A lymphocyte is shown at the left and a macrophage at the right. In particular, a subset of lymphocytes called T4 cells are infected; the hallmark of AIDS is a depletion of the T4 population. Unlike T4 cells, the macrophage is not killed by HIV. It may serve as a reservoir for the virus. The macrophage may also carry HIV to the brain, thereby accounting for the nervous-system pathology seen in AIDS.

marker for the T4 cells, it is also found in smaller numbers on some macrophages, allowing them to be infected.)

Several additional findings rounded out the early discoveries. The potential of the epidemic to spread beyond the original risk groups was shown when Robert R. Redfield and one of us (Gallo) demonstrated that HIV can be transmitted during heterosexual intercourse. Members of the Gallo team also showed that the genetic makeup of the virus is highly variable from strain to strain, a fact that may complicate the attempt to formulate an AIDS vaccine.

After the rapid initial advance the pace slowed somewhat and began to approximate that of a more mature area of research. Yet the continuing work was not without surprises. In October, 1985, one of us (Montagnier) was engaged in analyzing blood samples brought to his laboratory by a visiting investigator from Portugal. Many of the samples were from people who had lived in Guinea-Bissau, a former Portuguese colony in West Africa. Among them were some people who had been diagnosed by Portuguese clinicians and investigators as having AIDS in spite of the fact that their blood showed no sign of HIV infection.

One sample, in fact, was negative for HIV using the most sophisticated techniques available at the time. Yet workers in the laboratory were able to isolate a virus from the patient's blood. DNA "probes" (short pieces of DNA from the HIV genome) were then prepared. If the new virus were

closely related to the original AIDS agent, those probes would bind to its genetic material. As it turned out, there was little binding, and it became clear that the new isolate was not simply a strain of the original AIDS virus but a new virus designated HIV-2. Soon a second example was isolated by workers at the Claude Bernard Hospital; many others followed.

In evolutionary terms HIV-2 is clearly related to HIV-1, the virus responsible for the main AIDS epidemic. The two viruses are similar in their overall structure and both can cause AIDS, although the pathogenic potential of HIV-2 is not as well established as that of the first AIDS virus. HIV-2 is found mainly in West Africa, whereas HIV-1 is concentrated in central Africa and other regions of the world. The finding of HIV-2 suggests that other undiscovered HIV's may exist, filling out a spectrum of related pathogens.

The isolation of HIV-2 immediately raises the question of the evolutionary origins of these viruses (see Chapter 3, "The Origins of the AIDS Virus," by Max Essex and Phyllis J. Kanki). Although the answer to that question has not been found, some hints have been provided by the discovery in other primate species of related viruses called simian immunodeficiency viruses (SIV's). The first such virus, found in the macaque monkey, is designated SIV macaque. Isolated and characterized by Ronald C. Desrosiers and his co-workers at the New England Regional Primate Research Center in collaboration

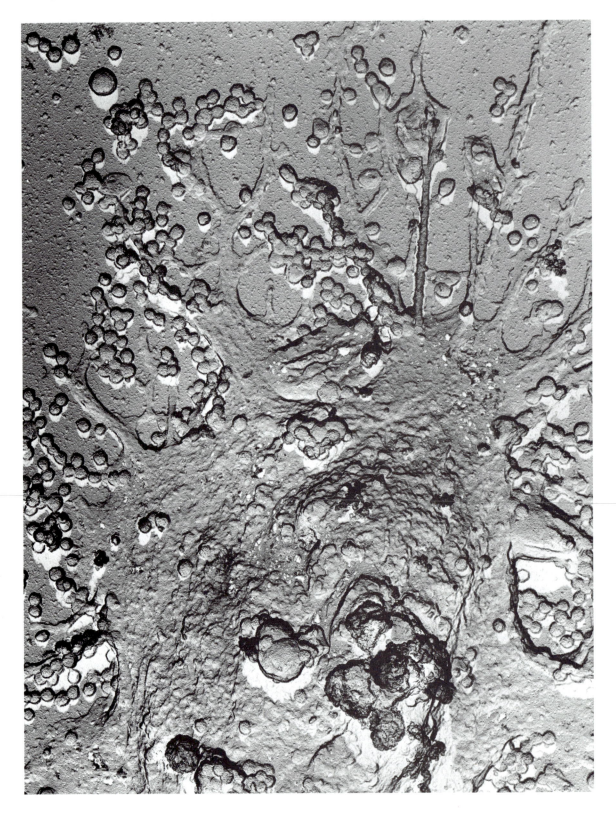

with Essex and his colleague Phyllis J. Kanki, SIV macaque has been shown to be closely related to HIV-2, raising the possibility that HIV-2 may have come into human beings relatively recently from another primate species.

No such close simian relative has been found for HIV-1 (although the right group of primates may not yet have been studied in sufficient detail). Hence the origin of HIV-1 remains more mysterious than the origin of its relative HIV-2. It is likely, however, that HIV-1 has been in human beings for some time. One of us (Gallo), with Temin, has used the divergence among HIV strains and the virus's probable rate of mutation to estimate how long the virus has infected people. It was tentatively concluded that HIV has infected human beings for more than 20 years but less than 100, an estimate compatible with those by other workers and with our knowledge of the epidemic.

Where was HIV hiding all those years, and why are we only now experiencing an epidemic? Both of us think the answer is that the virus has been present in small, isolated groups in central Africa or elsewhere for many years. In such groups the spread of HIV might have been quite limited and the groups themselves may have had little contact with the outside world. As a result the virus could have been contained for decades.

That pattern may have been altered when the way of life in central Africa began to change. People migrating from remote areas to urban centers no doubt brought HIV with them. Sexual mores in the city were different from what they had been in the village, and blood transfusions were commoner. Consequently HIV may have spread freely. Once a pool of infected people had been established, transport networks and the generalized exchange of blood products would have carried it to every corner of the world. What had been remote and rare became global and common (see Chapter 5, "The International Epidemiology of AIDS," by Jonathan M. Mann, James Chin, Peter Piot and Thomas Quinn).

Figure 6 SURFACE-REPLICA PREPARATION reproduces an infected cell and HIV particles. Such a preparation is made by dehydrating the cell, freeze-drying it and applying thin layers of platinum and carbon to its surface. The resulting replica is cleaned with acid, washed and examined in the electron microscope. The virus is distributed at the periphery of the cell and as free particles. (Micrograph, which has a magnification of about 40,000 diameters, by Gelderblom's colleague Muhsin Özel.)

What weapons are available against this scourge? Perhaps the best weapon is knowledge. One key form of knowledge is a deeper understanding of HIV, its life cycle and the mechanisms by which it causes disease. Although HIV kills T4 cells directly, it has become clear that the direct killing of those cells is not sufficient to explain the depletion seen in AIDS. Indirect mechanisms must also be at work. What are they?

Many possibilities have been suggested. Infection by HIV can cause infected and uninfected cells to fuse into giant cells called syncytia, which are not functional. Autoimmune responses, in which the immune system attacks the body's own tissues, may also be at work. What is more, HIV-infected cells may send out protein signals that weaken or destroy other cells of the immune system. In addition HIV is fragile, and as the virus particle leaves its host cell, a molecule called gp120 frequently falls off the virus's outer coat. As Dani P. Bolognesi of the Duke University Medical Center and his co-workers have shown, gp120 can bind to the CD4 molecules of uninfected cells. When that complex is recognized by the immune system, cells thus marked may be destroyed.

That list does not exhaust the possibilities. One of us (Montagnier) is exploring the possibility that the binding of the virus to its target cells triggers the release of enzymes called proteases. Proteases digest proteins, and if they were released in abnormal quantities, they might weaken white blood cells and shorten their lives. The various proposed mechanisms are not exclusive, and several may operate at once. Yet one is probably central, and some of the most significant work on AIDS is that of distinguishing the central mechanism from the peripheral ones that accompany it.

Although it is clear that a large enough dose of the right strain of HIV can cause AIDS on its own, cofactors can clearly influence the progression of the disease. People whose immune systems are weakened before HIV infection may progress toward AIDS more quickly than others; stimulation of the immune system in response to later infections may also hasten disease progression.

Interaction with other pathogens may also increase the likelihood that AIDS will develop. Specifically, a herpes virus called human B-cell lymphotropic virus (HBLV) or human herpes virus 6 (HHV-6) that was discovered in the laboratory of one of us (Gallo) can interact with HIV in a way that may increase the severity of HIV infection. Ordinarily HHV-6 is easily controlled by the immune system.

In a person whose immune system is impaired by HIV, however, HHV-6 may replicate more freely, becoming a threat to health. In addition, although one of the main hosts of HHV-6 is a white blood cell called the B cell, the virus can also infect T4 lymphocytes. If the T cell is simultaneously infected by HIV, HHV-6 can activate the latent AIDS virus, further impairing the immune system and worsening the cycle.

Clearly, in spite of rapid progress there are many gaps in our understanding of HIV and AIDS. Should we panic? The answer is no, for several reasons. The most obvious is that panic does no good. The second reason is that it now seems unlikely HIV infection will spread as rapidly outside the original high-risk groups in the industrial countries as it has within them. A third reason is that this disease is not beyond the curative power of science. Although current knowledge is imperfect, it is sufficient to provide confidence that effective therapies and a vaccine will be developed.

The possibilities for therapy are particularly impressive (see Chapter 8, "AIDS Therapies," by Robert Yarchoan, Hiroaki Mitsuya and Samuel Broder). In the first phase of the search for AIDS therapies it was necessary to exploit any drug that seemed to provide even a remote chance of combating HIV infection. A variety of compounds formulated for other purposes were taken off the shelf and tested. Most were of little value, but one (AZT), originally formulated as an anticancer drug, turned out to be the first effective anti-AIDS agent. More recently, an experimental regimen in which AZT is alternated with the related compound known as dideoxycytidine offers even greater promise.

Bringing AZT into clinical use was a significant accomplishment, because it gave hope that AIDS would not remain incurable forever. As a form of therapy, however, AZT is not perfect and will probably be supplanted by less toxic agents formulated on the basis of what is known about the HIV life cycle. One promising agent is CD4, the molecule that serves as the viral receptor. Early tests show that soluble CD4 can bind to the virus and prevent it from infecting new cells. Many other drugs are in trials; one of them, perhaps combined with compounds that bolster the immune system, may provide therapy for HIV infection.

In assessing the progress that has been made toward achieving fully effective AIDS therapy, it must be kept in mind that this work has two facets.

In addition to combating a complex and evasive pathogen, it must pioneer entirely new areas of medicine. The reason is that there are few effective treatments for viral diseases—and almost none for retroviruses. There are various reasons for this, among them the fact that viruses (unlike bacteria, for which effective therapies exist) always appropriate the biosynthetic apparatus of the host cell. As a result drugs effective against viruses tend to damage mammalian cells. Yet we are confident that the dual goals of pioneering science and clinical effectiveness will be met.

What is true of therapy is also true of vaccines: an AIDS vaccine will be a pioneering scientific achievement (see Chapter 9, "AIDS Vaccines," by Thomas J. Matthews and Dani P. Bolognesi). Since the HIV genome has the capacity to integrate into the chromosomes of the host cell, little serious consideration has been given to using preparations containing the whole virus as a vaccine. An AIDS vaccine must consist of subunits, or parts, of the virus in the right combination. Yet experience with subunit vaccines is slight. Indeed, so far only a few subunit vaccines have proved practical. Much work is under way to find the combination of HIV subunits that will yield the greatest protective response. As in the case of therapy, we believe there will be a practical vaccine against HIV.

Perhaps an even more persuasive reason for hope is that even without a vaccine or a cure, what is already known could bring the epidemic under control. The blood supply has already been largely secured by the presence of a blood test. Moreover, the modes of transmission of HIV—blood, sexual intercourse and from mother to child—are firmly established. Hence any individual can drastically reduce his or her risk of infection. If such knowledge were applied everywhere, there would be a sharp leveling off in the spread of HIV infection, as there has been in some groups in the developed world. The lesson here is that there is a need for education about HIV infection—in clear, explicit language and as early as possible.

Yet there are parts of the epidemic where education alone is not sufficient, and it is in those areas that humanity will be tested. Users of intravenous drugs, for example, are notoriously resistant to educational campaigns alone. It seems clear that the effort to control AIDS must be aimed in part at eradicating the conditions that give rise to drug addiction. Those conditions are in turn linked to social and economic patterns. Eliminating the disease may

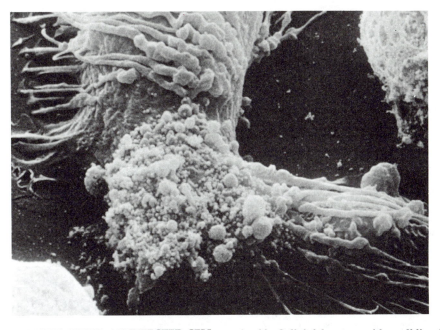

Figure 7 HIV PARTICLES COVER AN INFECTED CELL in culture. A central problem in obtaining specific reagents for establishing the cause of AIDS was that of getting HIV to grow in continuous mass culture. The problem was first solved in Gallo's laboratory with a cell line designated H9. An H9 cell is shown, magnified about 10,000 diameters. The small bumps at the center are HIV particles. (Micrograph by M. Özel.)

entail eliminating some of the social differentials that form the substratum of drug abuse (see Chapter 10, "The Social Dimensions of AIDS," by Harvey V. Fineberg).

It is also the case that in some areas of the developing world education alone will not stem the epidemic. Education is necessary, but it must be accompanied by other measures. In central Africa —the part of the world most beleaguered by AIDS— there are few facilities for blood testing and few technicians trained to perform tests. Furthermore, the blood tests used in the U.S. and Western Europe are too expensive to be helpful. As a result the virus is still being spread by contaminated blood, long after that form of transmission has been practically eliminated in the industrial countries.

To help change this situation the World AIDS Foundation has made improving the situation in central Africa its highest priority. The foundation (along with its parent, the Franco-American AIDS Foundation) was formed as part of the agreement that resolved a lawsuit between France and the U.S. over the AIDS blood test. The parent foundation receives 80 percent of the royalties from the French

and American blood tests; the World AIDS Foundation in turn receives 25 percent of that. Much thought has been given to how to allocate the funds, and the first project (carried out in conjunction with the World Health Organization) will be realized in several African countries. It will include training technicians to perform blood tests, establishing one HIV-free blood center and increasing public education about HIV transmission.

Efforts such as this one, coupling public and private funds and energies, will be essential to stopping AIDS. As we stated above, both of us are certain that science will ultimately find a cure and a vaccine for AIDS. But not tomorrow. The AIDS virus (and other human retroviruses) will be with us for a long time. During that time no intelligent person can expect the necessary solutions to come solely from authorities such as scientists, governments or corporations. All of us must accept responsibilities: to learn how HIV is spread, to reduce risky behavior, to raise our voices against acceptance of the drug culture and to avoid stigmatizing victims of the disease. If we can accept such responsibilities, the worst element of nightmare will have been removed from the AIDS epidemic.

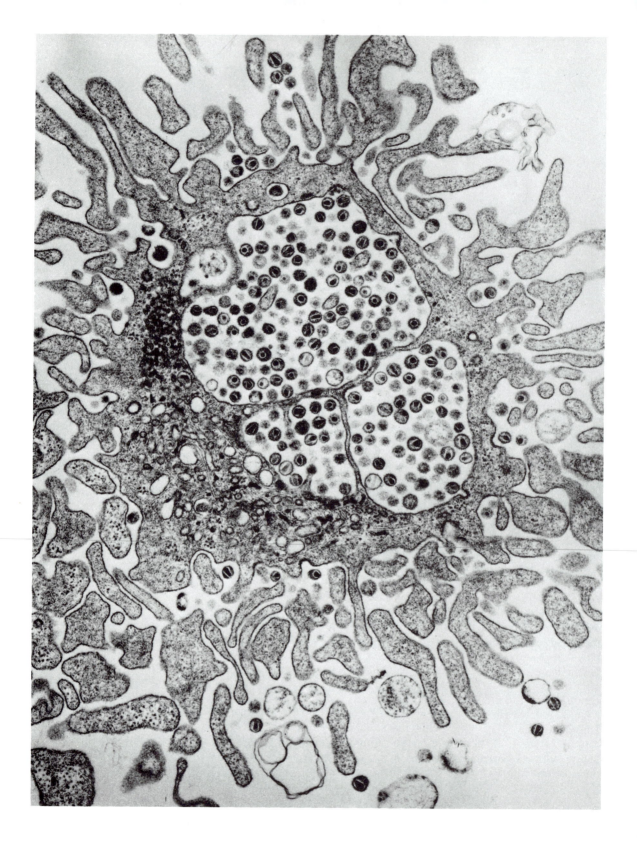

The Molecular Biology
of the AIDS Virus

HIV is genetically complex. An array of regulatory genes enables it to remain latent or replicate at various rates. This intricate control may underlie key features of the disease.

· · ·

William A. Haseltine and Flossie Wong-Staal

Infection with the AIDS virus takes many guises. First the virus (the human immunodeficiency virus, or HIV) often replicates abundantly, and free virus appears in the fluid surrounding the brain and spinal cord and in the bloodstream. Fevers, rashes, flulike symptoms and sometimes neurological complaints can accompany this first wave of HIV replication. Then, within a few weeks, the amount of virus in the circulation and the cerebro-spinal fluid drops precipitously and the initial symptoms disappear. Yet the virus is still present; it can be found not only in the T4 lymphocytes, the subset of immune-system cells originally thought to be its only target, but also in other classes of immune cells, in cells of the nervous system and intes-tine and probably in some bone-marrow cells. From two to 10 years after the start of this asymptomatic period, replication of the virus flares again and the infection enters its final stage.

Underlying this variable course are complex interactions between HIV and its host cells. The virus behaves differently depending on the kind of host cell and the cell's own level of activity. In T cells it can lie dormant indefinitely, inextricable from the cell but hidden from the victim's immune system; when the same cells are stimulated, however, it can destroy them in a burst of replication. In other cells, such as the immune-system cells called macrophages and their precursors, called monocytes, the virus grows continuously but slowly, sparing the cell but probably altering its function.

What accounts for this diverse behavior and its destructive consequences? The answer is to be found in the life cycle of the virus, and in the tiny package of genetic instructions that controls it. The genetic blueprint for the structure and life cycle of HIV is about 100,000 times smaller than the genetic information of a human cell: a mere 9,749 nucleotides (the units that encode information along the

Figure 8 CULMINATION of HIV's life cycle is the production of new virus. A cultured *T* cell is shedding newly formed virus particles, which are visible as small disks with a dark core. (Many particles have budded into vacuoles, enclosed sacs within the cell.) The viral genes that are responsible for the growth are emplaced in the nucleus of the infected cell. Magnification is about 25,000 diameters. (Micrograph by H. Gelderblom.)

genetic material). Since 1984, when HIV became available in a workable form, the full power of contemporary molecular biology and genetic analysis has been turned on this scrap of genetic information. The past four years have been full of surprises. HIV governs its life cycle in novel and unforeseen ways, and their study may hold the key not only to the control of AIDS but also to a clearer understanding of how cells regulate their own growth and activity.

In broadest outline the life cycle of HIV is that of a retrovirus. Retroviruses were so named because they reverse what seemed to be the normal flow of genetic information. In cells the genetic material is DNA; when genes are expressed, the DNA is first transcribed into messenger RNA (mRNA), which then serves as the template for the production of proteins. The genes of a retrovirus are encoded in RNA; before they can be expressed the RNA must be converted into DNA. Only then are the viral genes transcribed and translated into proteins in the usual sequence.

The cycle begins when an HIV particle binds to the outside of a cell and injects its core. The core includes two identical strands of RNA as well as structural proteins and enzymes that carry out later steps in the life cycle. One enzyme is responsible for converting the viral genetic information into DNA. This DNA polymerase first makes a single-strand DNA copy of the viral RNA. An associated enzyme, ribonuclease, destroys the original RNA, and the polymerase makes a second DNA copy, using the first one as a template. (The polymerase and the ribonuclease together are often called reverse transcriptase.)

The viral genetic information, now in the form of double-strand DNA (the same form in which the cell carries its own genes), migrates to the cell nucleus. A third viral enzyme, called an integrase, may then splice the HIV genome—its full complement of genetic information—into the host cell's DNA. Once there the viral DNA (the "provirus") will be duplicated together with the cell's own genes every time the cell divides. Thus established, infection is permanent.

The second half of the viral life cycle—the production of new virus particles—takes place only sporadically, and only in some infected cells. It begins when nucleotide sequences in the so-called long terminal repeats (LTR's), which are stretches of

DNA at the ends of the viral genome, direct enzymes belonging to the host cell to copy the DNA of the integrated virus into RNA. Some of the RNA will provide the genetic material for a new generation of virus. Certain other RNA strands serve as the mRNA's that guide cellular machinery in producing the structural proteins and enzymes of the new virus.

The particles, or virions, are assembled from multiple copies of two different protein molecules in a ratio of about 20 to one. The more abundant molecule is the precursor of the protein shell that will enclose the RNA and enzymes in the completed virions. The other molecule is larger; it contains the same structural components but includes additional segments that will become the viral enzymes. The two proteins migrate to the periphery of the cell as they are produced; a fatty acid at the end of each one attaches it to the inside of the cell membrane. As these precursors aggregate, they bind to one another and form a spherical structure that bulges outward under the cell membrane. Two strands of viral RNA are drawn into this nascent virion as it takes shape.

One of the enzymes contained in the longer precursor protein carries out the final step in producing mature virus. The enzyme, a protease (a protein-cleaving enzyme), cuts itself free of the protein chain and cleaves other enzymes (the DNA polymerase, ribonuclease and integrase, as well as additional molecules of protease) from long precursor molecules. It then divides the short precursors and what is left of the long ones into four segments each. Three of the segments collapse to form a bullet-shaped core surrounding the RNA and enzymes, but the remaining segment stays attached to the inside of the cell membrane.

Hence the completed virion encloses itself in a patch of host-cell membrane as it buds from the cell. This so-called envelope carries the final structural element of HIV: the envelope protein. The protein, which juts from the membrane like a set of minute spikes, is made and transported to the cell surface independently of the core proteins. Each spike is a complex of two or three identical units that in turn consist of two associated components. One component, called glycoprotein 120 (gp120) for its size and the fact that it is heavily glycosylated—coated with sugars—rests outside the cell and the other, gp41, is embedded stemlike in the membrane. These glycoprotein complexes, swept up by the budding virus as it acquires its

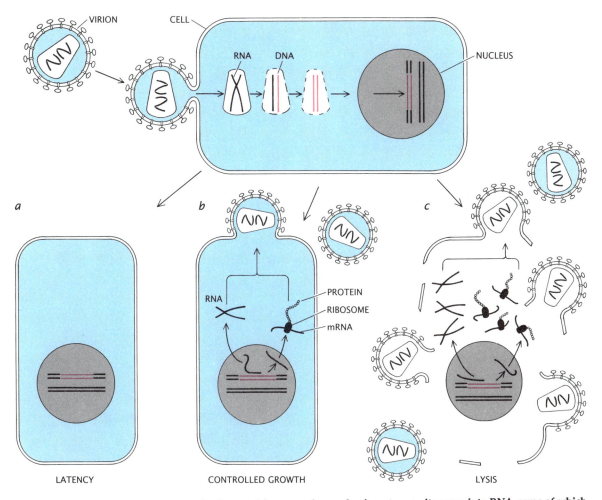

Figure 9 HIV INFECTION begins (*top*) **when a virion, or virus particle, binds to the outside of a susceptible cell and fuses with it, injecting the core proteins and two strands of viral RNA. The double-strand DNA (the "provirus") migrates to the nucleus and is integrated into the cell's own DNA. The provirus can then remain latent, giving no sign of its presence** (*a*). **Alternatively, it can commandeer cellular mechanisms to copy its genes into RNA, some of which is translated into viral proteins on structures called ribosomes. The proteins and additional RNA are then assembled into new virions that bud from the cell. The process can take place slowly, sparing the host cell** (*b*), **or so rapidly that the cell is lysed, or ruptured** (*c*).

envelope, are crucial to HIV's ability to infect new cells. (See Figures 3 and 10.)

An elaborate set of genetic controls determines whether this cycle of replication will be played out and how fast it will proceed. In addition to three genes for the proteins of the core and envelope, the HIV genome includes at least six other genes. Some and perhaps all of these genes act to regulate the production of viral proteins: one regulator speeds up protein synthesis generally, another speeds the production of only some kinds of proteins and a third gene represses protein synthesis. Since the regulatory genes themselves encode proteins, each one affects not only the structural genes but also the regulatory genes, including itself.

Their discovery, by our groups at the Dana-Farber Cancer Institute and the National Cancer Institute and by other workers, came as a surprise. The animal retroviruses that had been studied earlier have no such regulatory apparatus. In the early 1980's regulatory genes were found in the first two

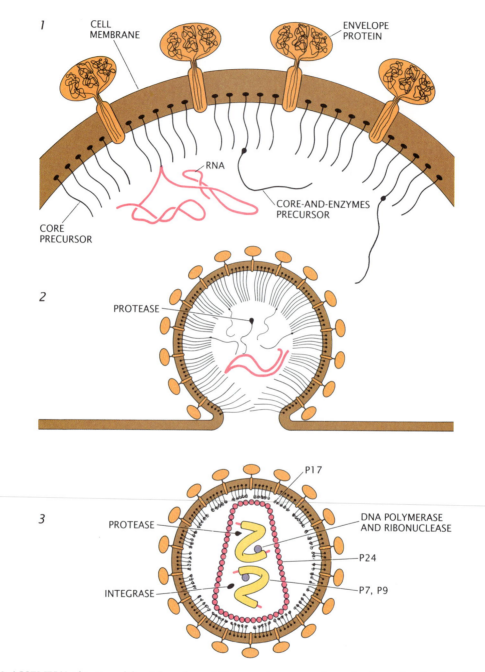

Figure 10 ASSEMBLY of a new virion takes place at the cell membrane. Three kinds of protein go into making the particle: the envelope protein and two precursor proteins of differing length (*1*). As the proteins aggregate at the cell membrane, it starts to pinch off. One precursor molecule draws two strands of viral RNA into the nascent virion, and a protease cuts itself free of a long precursor (*2*). The protease completes the formation by cleaving other enzymes from the long precursors and then cutting each of the precursors into four pieces. One piece (p17) remains attached to the patch of cell membrane that surrounds the completed particle, and the other three pieces (p24, p7 and p9) form a bullet-shaped inner core (*3*).

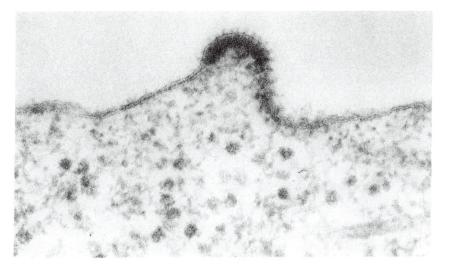

Figure 11 HIV BUDS from the surface of a cell. The particle is at the stage of assembly shown in Figure 10 (2); the envelope proteins studding the patch of cell membrane that will cloak the mature particle are visible in this electron micrograph, enlarged 120,000 diameters. (Image by H. Gelderblom.)

human retroviruses, the leukemia viruses HTLV-I and HTLV-II. But those discoveries did not foreshadow the number and complexity of HIV's regulatory pathways.

The pathways have been studied in part by observing the growth of virus in which one or another regulatory component has been inactivated by a mutation. Insight into the function of individual regulatory elements has also come from studying them in isolation: transferring them individually from HIV into the genetic material of experimental cell lines. Each regulatory gene encodes a protein that interacts specifically with a "responsive" element: a short sequence of nucleotides elsewhere in the genome. The regulatory protein is said to act in *trans*, because it exerts its effects at a distance; the responsive sequence affects adjacent genes and is said to act in *cis*. Individually or through their interplay the pathways can specify explosive viral replication, steady and moderate growth or quiescence.

A regulatory gene known as *tat*, for *trans*-activator, is responsible for the burst of replication seen, for example, in T4 cells that have been stimulated by an encounter with an antigen (a foreign molecule that evokes an immune response). The *tat* gene is unusual in both its structure and its effects. It is made up of two widely separated sequences of nu-

cleotides; after it is transcribed into mRNA the intervening genetic material must be spliced out before the transcript can be made into protein. The effect of the resulting small protein is dramatic: it can boost the expression of viral genes to 1,000 times the level seen in HIV mutants lacking the *tat* gene. The stimulatory effect extends to all the viral proteins, both the components of the virus particles and the regulatory proteins—including the *tat* protein itself. Because of this positive feedback, an enormous amount of virus is made very quickly when *tat* is activated.

To exert its effects the *tat* protein depends on a short sequence of nucleotides known as TAR (for *trans*-acting responsive sequence), which is found at the start of the viral genome and is included in the mRNA transcript of every HIV gene. Just how the protein and the TAR sequence interact is not clear, nor is it known how the interaction boosts protein synthesis. It has been proposed, variously, that *tat* and TAR increase the transcription of mRNA's from the viral DNA, the stability of completed mRNA's and the efficiency with which they are translated into proteins. The mechanism is not likely to be unique to HIV, and it is expected to shed light on the means by which higher organisms regulate gene expression.

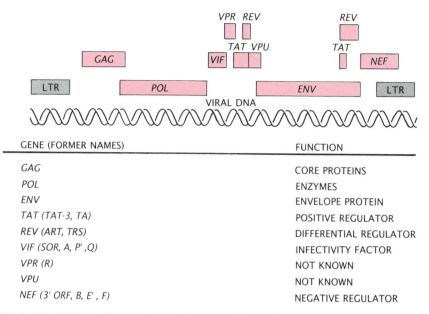

GENE (FORMER NAMES)	FUNCTION
GAG	CORE PROTEINS
POL	ENZYMES
ENV	ENVELOPE PROTEIN
TAT (TAT-3, TA)	POSITIVE REGULATOR
REV (ART, TRS)	DIFFERENTIAL REGULATOR
VIF (SOR, A, P', Q)	INFECTIVITY FACTOR
VPR (R)	NOT KNOWN
VPU	NOT KNOWN
NEF (3' ORF, B, E', F)	NEGATIVE REGULATOR

Figure 12 GENETIC STRUCTURE of HIV includes the nine genes identified so far, which are arranged along the viral DNA (*top*) and flanked by the long terminal repeats (LTR's). The LTR's, which do not code for any protein, serve to initiate the expression of other viral genes. Only three genes—*gag, pol* and *env*—encode components of virus particles; other genes serve to regulate the expression of these virion genes. Several regulatory genes are divided into noncontiguous pieces; the gene segments are spliced together in the RNA transcript from which protein is made. Because the DNA can be read in three ways, as many as three genes can coexist on one DNA segment.

Whereas *tat* boosts the production of viral proteins indiscriminately, a second regulatory gene, *rev*—the regulator of virion-protein expression—has differential effects. It enables the integrated virus to produce selectively either regulatory proteins or virion components. In addition to a *rev* protein, which like the *tat* product is encoded by noncontiguous nucleotide sequences that are spliced together in the mRNA, the *rev* pathway includes two other sequences. One of them prevents transcripts that include it from being turned into protein; the other sequence responds to the *rev* protein and overrides the first one's repressive effect.

The repression sequence is called the *cis*-acting repression element, or CRS. CRS sequences are built into the mRNA's that specify virion proteins: the core proteins, replication enzymes and envelope protein. The spliced, short mRNA's for regulatory proteins such as the *tat* protein and the *rev* protein itself lack the CRS sequence. In the absence of *rev*, the CRS sequence keeps the long mRNA templates for virion proteins from accumulating. Instead the truncated mRNA's that specify regulatory proteins, and that have had CRS spliced out, build up and are translated into protein.

The presence of the *rev* protein resets this genetic switch. The protein acts by way of a sequence called CAR—the *cis*-acting *rev*-responsive sequence, which like CRS is found in the long mRNA's—to counteract CRS. Full-length mRNA's now accumulate, and the production of regulatory proteins gives way to the production of proteins that make up a new generation of virus. In this way the *rev* pathway may control the shift from silent infection to active viral growth (see Figure 14).

Once replication is under way, however, interaction between the *rev* and *tat* mechanisms may hold viral growth in check. The two pathways can counteract each other: the *tat* product increases its own production and the production of the *rev* protein, whereas the *rev* protein slows its own synthesis and that of *tat* because it favors the accumulation of full-length mRNA's instead of the spliced mRNA's that form regulatory proteins. The result is a kind of homeostasis, marked by steady levels of both the *tat* and the *rev* proteins and modest production of virus. Because controlled growth enables a virus to reproduce itself for years without killing off its host cells, such genetic regulation may be an adaptive feature for any retrovirus that infects a long-lived species such as human beings. Indeed, the other human retroviruses, HTLV-I and -II, also have *tat*- and *rev*like controls.

How can a regulatory pathway alternately favor the synthesis of proteins from two different sets of genes? Results from a series of experiments suggest that the *rev* pathway does not directly affect the production of mRNA or protein. Instead it may act by governing the transport of mRNA's. This hypothesis assumes the existence of several subcompartments within the infected cell's nucleus; mRNA's would meet different fates depending on which subcompartment they were shunted into.

Under this hypothesis the CRS sequence ordinarily would interact with cellular transport mechanisms to confine the mRNA's it marks (the mRNA's for virion proteins) in a nuclear subcompartment that contains splicing mechanisms and powerful degradative enzymes. There the transcripts would be either spliced to remove the CRS sequences or degraded. Any spliced transcripts, which would now encode regulatory proteins, could then be exported from the nucleus to the protein factories in the cytoplasm of the cell.

If the *rev* protein is present, on the other hand, the CAR sequence would respond by overriding the CRS signal. Then full-length mRNA's would be shunted to a nuclear subcompartment in which they would escape splicing and degradation; from there they would be exported and made into virion proteins (see Figure 15). In view of this hypothesis it is noteworthy that the *rev* protein is distributed unevenly in the nucleus of HIV-infected cells, as one might expect it to be if it exerts its effect in a specific subcompartment.

In addition to an activator (*tat*) and a selective regulator (*rev*), HIV is equipped with a negative regulator, which slows the transcription of the viral genome. The gene is called *nef* (negative-regulatory factor), and it may be responsible for HIV's ability to turn off its own growth and lie utterly dormant. The *nef* protein's target sequence, found at the start of the viral genome in the long terminal repeat, is known as NRE (negative-regulatory element). The NRE sequence represses transcription even on its own; when the viral LTR is transferred into uninfected cells, it directs a higher rate of transcription of

cellular genes if it lacks the sequence. The *nef* product amplifies NRE's effect.

Just how the *nef* protein does so is a puzzle. In contrast to the *tat* and *rev* proteins, which are concentrated in the nucleus, close to the HIV genes they affect, the *nef* protein is found mainly outside the nucleus in the cytoplasm. Indeed, the molecule bears a fatty acid that probably locks it onto the inside of the cell membrane. How can this distant factor interact with the NRE sequence in the viral genome?

It is likely that the *nef* protein exerts its effect through intermediary molecules made by the host cell. The protein displays several activities similar to those of molecules that initiate or take part in the cell's own signaling pathways, which relay chemical messages received at the cell membrane to processes within the cell. For example, the biochemistry of the *nef* protein resembles the biochemistry of cellular agents that can trigger the activation of a protein kinase, a kind of enzyme that directly stimulates many cellular responses. In addition the *nef* protein is itself a protein kinase and can be modified by a cellular protein kinase. All these properties suggest that the *nef* protein acts by affecting cellular factors that ultimately carry its message to the NRE sequence in the nucleus (see Figure 16).

The repressive effect of *nef* is intertwined with the activities of the other regulatory pathways. The countervailing effects of the *nef* and *tat* pathways could lead to prolonged steady-state production of both proteins and controlled viral growth — a consequence similar to that of the interplay between *rev* and *tat*. The interaction of *nef* and *rev*, on the other hand, could foster instability and underlie HIV's characteristic extreme variations in growth rate.

Both pathways are negative-feedback loops. The *nef* protein slows its own production as well as the production of the *rev* product by suppressing transcription of all viral genes, whereas the *rev* protein achieves the same effects by slowing the production of regulatory proteins in favor of structural ones. The interaction holds the potential of an all-or-nothing response. A high initial concentration of the *nef* protein would suppress all further gene expression and the virus would lie quiescent; a high initial concentration of *rev* would suppress further production of regulatory proteins (including *nef*) in favor of structural ones. Viral replication would be switched on.

This picture of three regulatory pathways interacting to set the level of viral growth may soon be

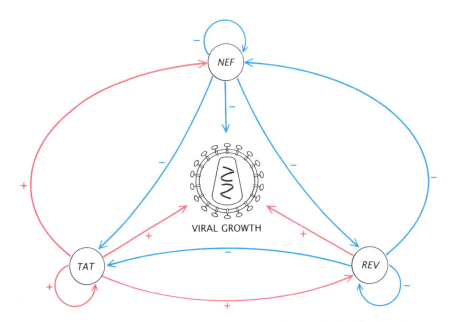

Figure 13 NETWORK OF INTERACTIONS among HIV regulatory genes controls viral growth. Each gene, through its protein product and the sequence in the viral genetic material that responds to it, affects the expression not only of the genes for virion components but also of the other regulatory genes and (in a feedback effect) itself. The *tat* gene acts by positive feedback and activates (*red arrows*) all HIV genes; *nef* acts by negative feedback and represses (*blue arrows*) all the genes. The *rev* gene represses regulatory genes but activates virion genes, favoring viral growth.

complicated further. HIV contains two newly identified genes, *vpr* and *vpu,* that are active in the course of infection. Perhaps the *vpr* and *vpu* products also regulate viral replication. Studies of these two proteins and their possible interactions with known regulatory factors are at an early stage, however.

These intricate mechanisms for controlling HIV growth do not operate in isolation; they are intimately intertwined with the physiology of the host cell. For one thing, the virus depends on cellular machinery to transcribe its genes and convert them into protein. More specifically, cellular factors surely contribute to the *tat*-driven burst of HIV replication that ensues when an infected *T* cell is stimulated by antigen. Differences in the host molecular climate must also play some part in the varied levels of growth seen in different cell types. What is the basis of these influences?

One key phenomenon may be the interaction of cellular proteins with the LTR at the beginning of the viral genome. Sequences in the LTR define the RNA initiation site: the starting point for the copying of

viral genes into mRNA. The sequences resemble those found at the initiation sites of cellular genes, and at least eight proteins that are normally engaged in cellular transcription bind to the viral genome at or near the initiation site. One probably serves to position the RNA polymerase (the cellular enzyme that copies genes into mRNA) as transcription begins, and several other proteins are believed to speed the rate of RNA initiation.

One protein that recognizes the HIV initiation sequences has a specific role in the physiology of *T* cells and other lymphocytes. The protein, designated NF-κB, is activated when lymphocytes are stimulated by an antigen and begin to multiply, and it is thought to contribute to cell growth by increasing transcription. It turns out that stimulation of infected *T* cells increases the binding of NF-κB to the viral genome. The activation of this protein, then, may be one means by which *T*-cell stimulation precipitates viral growth.

Not all the cellular proteins that act on the viral genome are stimulatory; some must repress gene expression. The virus's *nef* protein, for example, which acts from a distance to slow the expression of viral genes, relies on cellular intermediaries to carry its signal to the NRE sequence in the nucleus. That sequence's ability to slow transcription even in the absence of *nef*, moreover, probably reflects an independent interaction with inhibitory factors made by the cell.

The constellation of cellular factors acting on the viral genome presumably varies depending on both the condition and the kind of host cell. Some resting cells may simply lack the proteins needed for RNA initiation, so that the infection remains quiescent. In other cells the rate of viral growth may be constrained by a low concentration of initiation factors

or by an abundance of proteins that inhibit mRNA synthesis. Thus the host cell, through its array of transcription factors, creates a molecular environment that influences the working of HIV's own regulatory mechanisms.

After those mechanisms trigger the production of infectious virus particles, a final gene comes into play. Called *vif*, for virion infectivity factor, the gene encodes a small protein that is found in the cytoplasm of infected cells, in the fluid surrounding them and perhaps also in free virus particles. The *vif* protein somehow enhances the ability of virus that

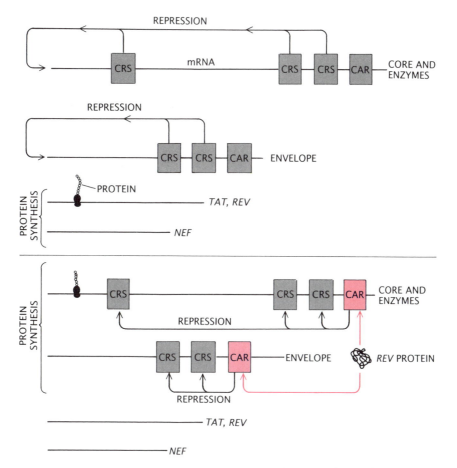

Figure 14 GENETIC SWITCH for viral growth is embodied in the *rev* pathway. The pathway includes two nucleotide sequences designated CRS and CAR, which are found in the messenger RNA's (mRNA's) for components of the virus core and envelope. In the absence of *rev* protein (*top*), CRS represses the synthesis of protein from these mRNA's, and the elements of new virus are not made. Only the short mRNA's for regulatory proteins (the *rev*, *tat* and *nef* products), which lack CRS, are made into protein. When the *rev* protein is present (*bottom*), it interacts with CAR to override the repressive effect of CRS; virion proteins are made and viral growth is switched on.

has budded from one cell to infect another; HIV strains carrying mutations that inactivate *vif* make normal-looking virions that carry a full complement of RNA and enzymes but infect cells less efficiently.

In the absence of *vif* the initial step in infection occurs just as readily: gp120, the outer part of the envelope protein that studs the virion surface, binds to a specific protein on the surface of an uninfected cell. This receptor molecule, known as CD4, is abundant on the surface of *T*4 cells but is also present in at least trace amounts on every kind of cell infected by the virus (see Chapter 7, "HIV Infection: The Cellular Picture," by Jonathan N. Weber and Robin A. Weiss).

Next, in the ordinary course of events, one end of gp41, the part of the envelope protein that is embedded in the viral membrane, pierces the membrane of the target cell and initiates fusion. (An unidentified cell-surface component known as fusion factor, the absence of which prevents infection of certain cell lines even though they are rich in CD4, must also be present.) The core of the virus then enters the cell, and the viral genome is copied into DNA and integrated in the cell nucleus.

In *vif*-defective virus one of these later steps apparently takes place very inefficiently. The absence of the *vif* product hampers only the transmission of free virus, however. The virus can still spread by cell-to-cell transmission, in which viral envelope protein on the surface of an infected cell binds to the CD4 receptor on an uninfected cell and the cell membranes fuse, allowing virus cores that have formed but not yet budded from the infected cell to pass into the new cell and infect it.

What is the molecular basis for the cellular devastation that accompanies this intricately controlled cycle of growth and dissemination? HIV infection practically eliminates the entire population of *T*4 cells and may also kill their precursors in the thymus gland and the bone marrow. It does so even though the number of infected *T* cells at any given time is quite low. Moreover, the virus is just as common in other cell populations, such as macrophages and monocytes, and yet it kills relatively few of those cells.

The properties of the viral envelope protein explain much of this pattern of cell death. The envelope protein kills cells directly in at least two ways. As virus particles bud from an infected cell, the protein on the departing virus may bind to CD4 molecules on the surrounding cell membrane, tear-

ing holes in it. The punctured cell swells and dies. Prolific viral replication and a high concentration of surface CD4 are both needed for this means of killing cells. Infected *T* cells meet both criteria; infected macrophages, monocytes and microglial cells (structural cells in the brain and spinal cord) produce virus slowly and display little CD4. They generally escape destruction by this mechanism.

The envelope protein can also kill *T* cells in quantity by another means: the same process of cell fusion that is responsible for cell-to-cell transmission of the virus. Beginning with a single infected cell, the process of fusion, mediated by gp120 and the CD4 molecule, can continue until as many as 500 uninfected cells have combined into a giant, moribund mass called a syncytium. The ability of this process to multiply the cell-killing effect of infection may explain how *T*4 cells become drastically depleted in AIDS patients even though at any given instant fewer than one in every 1,000 *T* cells harbors the virus in active or latent form.

In a third process of cell killing, carried out by the immune system itself, the envelope protein has an indirect role. The immune system of a person infected with HIV makes antibodies to the envelope protein as well as to other viral proteins, yet this immune response does not eliminate or inactivate the virus. Important functional sites on the envelope protein, in particular, seem to be mostly protected from antibodies by its shape, its shroud of sugar molecules and the continual variation that results from mutations in the gene encoding it (see Chapter 9, "AIDS Vaccines," by Thomas J. Matthews and Dani P. Bolognesi).

Not only does the immune response to the envelope protein fail to check the disease but also it may be fatal to the patient's own cells — cells such as macrophages and monocytes, which HIV does not kill directly. Antibodies that have bound to the envelope protein (routinely displayed on infected cells) may activate a set of blood proteins known as complement, which lyses, or ruptures, the antibody-coated cells. A subset of lymphocytes known as killer *T* cells may also respond to the envelope protein by destroying infected cells. The viral protein could make even uninfected cells into targets for immune-mediated killing. Infected cells readily shed gp120; the free protein can then bind to CD4 on healthy cells, subjecting them to attack by agents of the immune system.

The envelope protein is the only HIV component whose role in cell killing has been documented. Yet

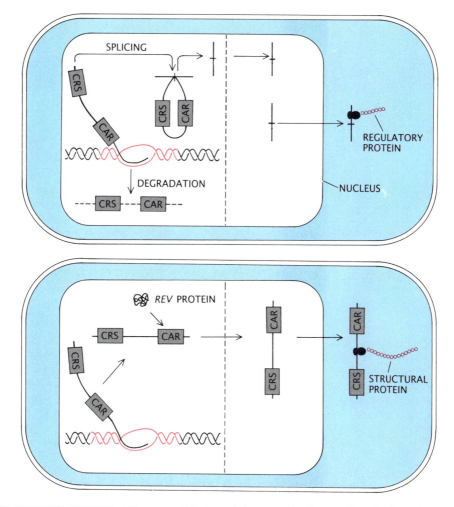

Figure 15 POSSIBLE MECHANISM of the *rev* switch depends on the selective transport of mRNA's. In the absence of the *rev* protein (*top*) any mRNA's that include the CRS sequence are held in the nucleus in a hypothetical subcompartment, where they are either degraded or spliced to remove CRS. Spliced transcripts can then be transported into a second subcompartment, where they are stable, and ultimately made into protein; because of the splicing, however, they yield only regulatory proteins. The *rev* protein interacts with CAR to override CRS (*bottom*). Full-length mRNA's can now be transported into the second subcompartment and then made into virion proteins.

the regulatory proteins may also contribute to cell death or dysfunction, by altering the expression of cellular as well as viral genes. The *nef* protein, for example, relying as it does on cellular factors to carry its message of repression to the viral genome, is very likely to have broader effects on the cell; *tat*, *rev* and perhaps other HIV genes may also disturb the cell's genetic control. Among the cellular genes thus affected might be those that direct the production of diffusible factors that help to maintain immune-system function.

For example, macrophages and monocytes release protein factors, such as interleukin-1 and interferons, that activate other cell populations in the immune system. Abnormally high or low levels of these factors could alter the behavior of the target cells or even kill them. Cells in the central nervous system require similar diffusible proteins for their survival, which raises the possibility that altered macrophage and monocyte function underlies some of the neurological deterioration seen in AIDS patients.

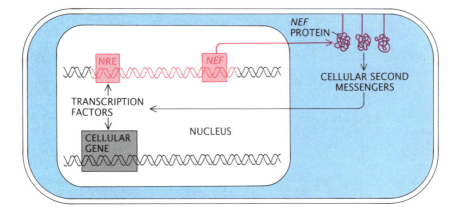

Figure 16 ACTION AT A DISTANCE characterizes the *nef* **pathway, which represses HIV growth. The protein encoded by** *nef* **is found in the cell cytoplasm, probably attached to the inside of the cell membrane. Yet it seems to exert its effects by way of NRE, a sequence in the viral genome, in the nucleus. It is thought that cellular signaling systems and factors probably carry the** *nef* **protein's message to the nucleus. By affecting the cell's own biochemistry,** *nef* **might also alter the expression of cellular genes.**

The viral genetic blueprint that specifies these events, from infection through replication to cell killing, is remarkably changeable. The complete sequence of nucleotides has been determined for a number of HIV samples, isolated at different times and places. Some pairs of isolates differ in no more than 1 or 2 percent of their nucleotides, but for other isolates the differences amount to more than 25 percent. What is the source of this striking variability?

HIV replication includes three steps at which mutations are likely. The viral DNA polymerase lacks the error-correcting feature that analogous cellular enzymes have, and so the copying errors it makes in converting viral RNA into a single DNA strand and then synthesizing the complementary strand go uncorrected. The cellular RNA polymerase that makes the genetic material for new virions also does not correct its own errors. These three steps are common to all retroviruses; in a bird retrovirus they — together with other, less problematic events in replication — have been found to produce an average of about one mutation per replication cycle.

At that rate new HIV variants can develop during a single infection. And yet if one sets aside differences in the disease's course and transmission properties that can be ascribed to environmental or social factors, AIDS shows a remarkably consistent face throughout the world. Why is the variability of the virus not reflected in the nature of the disease?

Many mutations leave HIV unable to survive and so are eliminated. The many other mutations that persist are concentrated in parts of the genome that are thought to have little functional role. Most mutations, then, are not likely to affect the structure and life cycle of the virus, and so strains that are rather different genetically may have similar pathogenic properties. In virus that has been maintained in culture, mutations do appear in the regulatory genes; such mutations can increase a cultured strain's growth rate by, for example, incapacitating the negative-regulatory gene *nef*. Yet mutations affecting genetic regulation do not seem common in natural infections; nearly all patients make antibodies to the *nef* protein, for instance.

That is not to say that mutations play no role at all in the pathology of AIDS. The advent of variants carrying mutations in the envelope gene in particular may well affect the progression of the disease in an individual. Changes in an exposed part of the envelope protein called the hypervariable loop, for example, may enable the virus to evade an immune response directed at the protein and so would be favored by natural selection. Mutational change in other parts of the protein may alter the virus's ability to bind to or fuse with a specific kind of cell. As one population of cells becomes depleted, HIV variants with an increased affinity for another cell population might have the advantage.

This is the molecular character of the opponent facing clinicians and workers in drug and vaccine development. The picture is a daunting one. HIV is able to slip into cells and remain there for life. Its elaborate genetic regulation enables it to lie low, hidden from immune surveillance; to replicate slowly, possibly deranging the host cell's own genetic controls as it does so, or to initiate a burst of growth that kills the infected cell. Even when HIV is active, the design of its envelope protein and the variability that results from its error-prone replication mechanisms make it a difficult target for an immune response.

A molecular description of HIV, then, reveals the full dimensions of the challenge presented by AIDS. Yet it also sets out the vital features of the virus, some of which can serve as the focus of control strategies. Surely this description contains the seeds of HIV's eventual defeat.

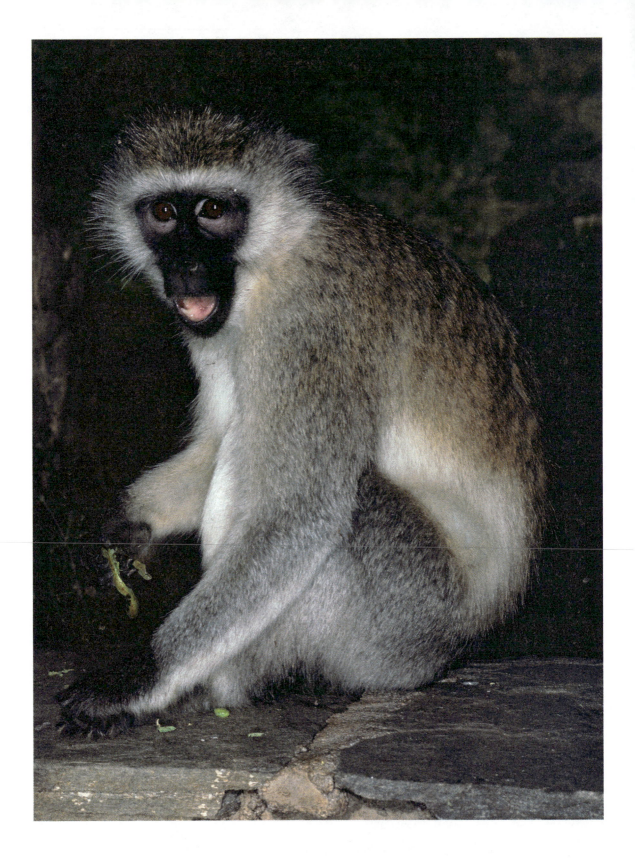

The Origins of the AIDS Virus

The AIDS virus is not unique. It has relatives in man as well as other primates. Studies of related viruses indicate that some have evolved disease-free coexistence with their animal hosts.

• • •

Max Essex and Phyllis J. Kanki

The sudden appearance and rapid spread of a previously unknown infectious disease such as AIDS raises a series of compelling questions. What is the causative agent, what is its structure and how does it function and — in the case of a previously unknown agent — where did it come from?

Our own work has addressed the third problem, that of the origin of the AIDS virus, HIV. The object of these studies, we should make clear, is not to identify a particular site or group of people that harbored a particular ancestral virus and trace a path that led to the AIDS pandemic. Rather, the object is to learn more about viruses related to HIV and so understand how HIV has evolved the unique and deadly properties that lead to AIDS.

These questions are of more than historical interest. Within the past three years we and others have identified retroviruses related to HIV in monkeys and in human beings. The different biological properties of the viruses in various hosts can reveal something about how they cause disease. Evolutionary selection tends in the long run to favor the survival of both a virus and its host. Over decades or millenniums a virus-host relation can change; a lethal disease caused by a virulent pathogen in a susceptible host tends to give way as less virulent viruses and more resistant hosts emerge. Understanding how this may have happened in the case of other viruses may reveal ways to control the AIDS virus and its disease.

One way to begin searching out the origin of HIV is to look for similar viruses in nonhuman primates. Monkeys and apes are often the only animal species other than human beings that are infected with important human viruses such as yellow fever and Marburg virus; in certain cases it is even thought that wild monkeys harbor the pathogens and can be the source of human infections.

The search for monkey viruses related to HIV had a precedent in the discovery of a primate counterpart of another human retrovirus. The first retroviruses shown to infect human beings (in 1980, by Robert C. Gallo of the National Cancer Institute)

Figure 17 AFRICAN GREEN MONKEY is a major reservoir of the simian immunodeficiency virus (SIV), a relative of the AIDS virus; in various green-monkey populations from 30 to 70 percent of the animals are infected. Yet SIV does not cause disease in the infected green monkeys — whereas it causes simian AIDS in, for example, Asian macaques in primate research centers. Why?

were two human *T*-lymphotropic viruses: HTLV-I (the cause of a rare form of *T*-cell leukemia/lymphoma in people) and the very closely related HTLV-II. Two years later Isao Miyoshi of Kochi University described a related virus in a monkey, the Japanese macaque. The virus was remarkably similar to the HTLV's and was designated the simian *T*-lymphotropic virus, STLV.

Both the HTLV's and STLV were capable of inducing immortality (one characteristic of cells transformed to the cancerous state) in *T* lymphocytes grown in the laboratory. The proteins of the two types of viruses were very similar: antibodies elicited by either virus in its host could recognize the proteins of the other virus—a phenomenon known as cross-reactivity. The genetic material of STLV was organized much like that of HTLV and the sequence of its component nucleotides was between 90 and 95 percent homologous to, or identical with, that of HTLV. Besides these virological similarities, the monkey and human viruses had similar biological properties.

When we studied Asian macaques at the New England Regional Primate Research Center in Southborough, Mass., we found that monkeys with malignant lymphoma (a cancer of lymphoid cells) showed much higher rates of STLV infection than healthy macaques. It appeared, then, that STLV was capable of inducing a lymphoid cancer in monkeys similar to the HTLV-induced lymphoid cancer in people.

The discovery of STLV prompted a number of studies aimed at determining its distribution in various primate species worldwide; the hope was to find clues to the geographic and evolutionary origin of HTLV. The simian virus was found to infect both Asian and African Old World monkeys and apes; in various serological studies (in which blood samples are analyzed for the presence of specific antibodies) the rate of STLV infection in these species varied from 1 to 40 percent. Genetic studies of STLV's from Asian and African primates showed that the human virus was more closely related to the simian virus seen in the African chimpanzee or the African green monkey (95 percent homology) than to the virus seen in the Asian macaque (90 percent), indicating that African STLV might have played the more important role in the origin and evolution of human HTLV's.

One hypothesis regarding the origin of HTLV relied on the premise that the 5 percent difference in the genetic sequences of the African STLV and

HTLV was so great that it ruled out any possibility of a monkey-virus transfer to human beings any time after New World primates diverged from the Old World primate lineage during the Eocene epoch, about 40 million years ago. HTLV, then, would have evolved very long ago, from a virus infecting the primate ancestor that gave rise to the great apes.

If that were the case, however, the parallel evolution of STLV and HTLV within their respective hosts would need to have been virtually identical, considering that at the present time the two viruses differ by less than 5 percent. Many of us thought it unlikely that retroviruses could maintain such similarity after millions of years of evolution in various host species that were themselves evolving.

This suggested that primates could have infected human beings with a version of STLV in more recent times, within the past 40 million years. Indeed, Gallo has proposed that HTLV originated in Africa, where both people and African primates were infected, and was spread to the Americas by the slave trade and to the southwestern islands of Japan (the virus's other endemic area) by oceangoing Portuguese traders. Regardless of just how STLV and HTLV entered their respective host species, the available data made it clear that their origins were inextricably linked.

This background provided the impetus, after the AIDS virus had been characterized, for us to undertake a search for a monkey virus related to HIV. In 1984 we set about examining large numbers of primates by serological testing. Any virus infecting these primates that was related to HIV would share with HIV some sites (called cross-reactive epitopes) on its viral proteins. When an HIV-related protein was present in an infected animal, it would elicit cross-reactive antibodies to these epitopes, and we could detect the antibodies in the monkeys' blood. Soon we succeeded in finding such antibodies—

Figure 18 PRIMATES AND RETROVIRUSES that infect them are related as shown. (The diagram is not drawn to reflect the precise sequence or dating of the evolutionary branching.) STLV, the first monkey retrovirus discovered, is not seen in New World monkeys; presumably it originated after they diverged from the main primate lineage. SIV infects African green monkeys in the wild. The hatched symbols indicate primate species that have been infected experimentally. HIV-1 and HIV-2 infect humans and, in the laboratory, certain primates.

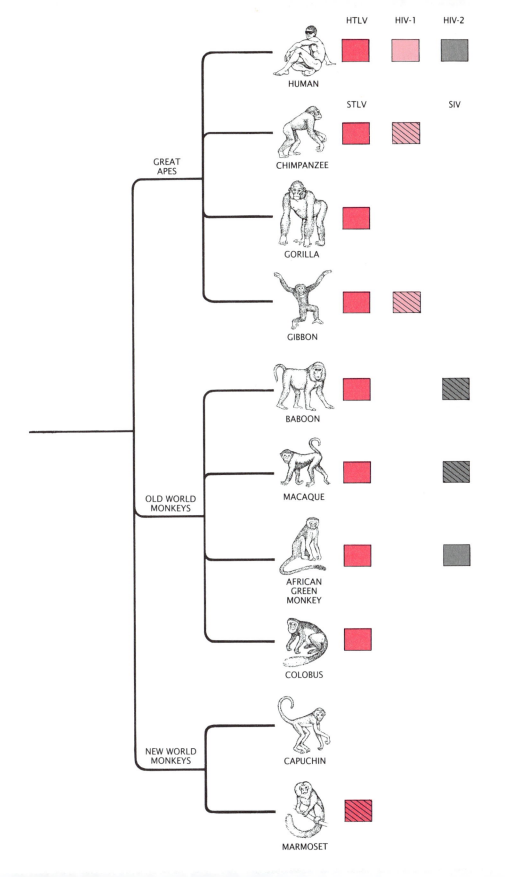

and hence evidence for the presence of a monkey virus related to HIV—in blood samples from Asian macaques (*Macaca* spp.) housed at the New England primate center.

At about that time veterinary pathologists at several primate research centers in the U.S. were reporting outbreaks of AIDS-like disease in captive macaque monkeys. The illness (called SAIDS, for simian AIDS) was seen only in Asian macaques. We were able to identify HIV-related antibodies in the SAIDS macaques. Then, in collaboration with Norman L. Letvin, Ronald C. Desrosiers and Muthiah D. Daniel of the New England center, we isolated and characterized the virus infecting them, which is now designated the simian immunodeficiency virus (SIV).

It was clearly related to HIV, as the antibody studies had suggested it would be. It infected the same CD4 subset of lymphocytes the human virus infects. The biochemical and biophysical properties of the SIV proteins were very similar to those of the HIV proteins. Antibodies from AIDS patients recognized cross-reactive epitopes on the SIV proteins, just as the monkey antibodies had recognized HIV proteins. The human antibodies were highly reactive with the major core protein of SIV but only minimally cross-reactive with the envelope glycoproteins on the surface of the monkey virus. It is characteristic of retroviruses that the internal core proteins are the most conserved, or "group-specific": they tend to be common to the members of a group of viruses. The envelope glycoproteins, on the other hand, are the least conserved—they are more "type-specific," or distinct for each virus in the group.

Subsequent genetic studies have shown that SIV is approximately 50 percent related to HIV at the nucleotide-sequence level. The organization of structural and regulatory genes is virtually identical in SIV and HIV. The notable exceptions are the *vpx* gene of SIV, which is not found in HIV, and the *vpu* gene of HIV, which is not found in SIV. Like humans infected with HIV, Asian macaques infected with SIV suffered a decrease in *T4* lymphocytes with ensuing immunosuppression; the animals died of opportunistic infections very similar to those seen in human AIDS. These features of SIV provide striking parallels to those of HIV. SIV therefore represents a system in which drugs and vaccines aimed at HIV can be subjected to preliminary testing.

As we studied SIV in 1985, the similarities between the simian virus and the human virus suggested that the two must be related, and we wondered whether the geographic distribution of the monkey virus might provide clues to the origin of the human AIDS virus. The mere existence of a related virus in captive immunosuppressed monkeys maintained in a U.S. primate facility did not provide much information in that respect. The monkey virus could have been transmitted to the macaques from another monkey species housed in the same facility or even by experimental manipulations.

We therefore investigated the possibility that wild Asian macaques also harbored SIV. Seroepidemiological studies of wild and captive Asian monkeys, including macaques, failed to find evidence of an SIV- or HIV-like agent. Studies by many investigators confirmed that SIV infection in the Asian macaque was limited to small numbers of monkeys in captivity, where it was highly associated with SAIDS. The data suggested that SIV did not naturally infect Asian monkeys in the wild. It seemed quite possible that the primate-center macaques had been exposed to SIV in captivity.

If the Asian macaque monkey was not the natural host for SIV, then what was? And how (if at all) were the primate viruses related to the observed emergence of HIV in people? In 1985 the highest rates of HIV were reported in the U.S. and Europe, but disturbing reports from central Africa indicated that high rates of HIV infection and of AIDS prevailed there, at least in some urban centers. The reported rates of infection were so high that many workers thought the AIDS epidemic in central Africa might have predated the emergence of the disease elsewhere in the world. On the assumption that the distribution of HIV in human populations might be correlated with the distribution of related viruses in monkeys, it seemed to us to be important to determine whether HIV-related viruses were present in primate species in Africa.

We therefore obtained blood samples from representative African primates, including wild-caught chimpanzees (*Pan troglodytes*), African green monkeys (*Cercopithecus aethiops*), baboons (*Papio spp.*) and patas monkeys (*Erythrocebus patas*). The samples were analyzed for the presence of antibodies that reacted with proteins of the SIV virus from macaques. We found no evidence of SIV infection in the chimpanzee, baboon or patas monkey—but more than 50 percent of the wild African green monkeys studied in our first survey did show evidence of an SIV infection.

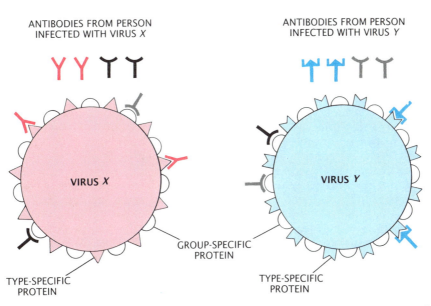

Figure 19 CROSS-REACTIVITY is displayed by related viruses. Each virus has on its surface type-specific proteins that are uniquely its own and group-specific ones that it shares with related viruses. Some antigenic sites (epitopes) on group-specific proteins are common to both viruses. A person infected by virus X will have developed cross-reactive antibodies that recognize cross-reactive epitopes on related virus Y.

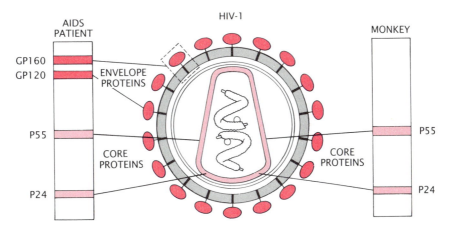

Figure 20 SIV was discovered by serological testing. AIDS patients have antibodies that recognize HIV-1 envelope proteins (gp120 and its precursor gp160) and core proteins (p24 and its precursor p55). Both Asian macaques that had simian AIDS and African green monkeys were found to have antibodies that recognized the HIV-1 core proteins (which are generally the more cross-reactive proteins in a retrovirus). The antibody response showed the monkeys had been infected with a virus related to HIV-1.

We have since analyzed samples from several thousand African green monkeys caught in various regions of sub-Saharan Africa and from many others housed in research facilities throughout the world. We find SIV infection in from 30 to 70 percent of them. Yet they show no sign of immunosuppression or of SAIDS. Moreover, in spite of their having the highest rates of SIV infection, the various green-monkey subspecies are among the most ecologically successful African primates, suggesting that the high infection rate in these monkeys has not been exerting long-term adverse selection pressure on the species.

Why SIV is endemic in these wild African monkeys but seems to do them no harm, and is also found in the captive Asian macaques, where it causes disease, was (and still is) an enigma, but the puzzle pointed to a line of investigation. It seemed quite possible that the captive Asian monkeys might first have been infected when they were accidentally exposed to African monkeys in holding facilities. The fact that a virus that seemed to be quite harmless in African monkeys was wreaking havoc in the newly exposed Asian monkeys indicated that at least some strains of SIV still had a potential for great virulence. The infected African species must have evolved mechanisms that kept a potentially lethal pathogen from causing disease. Indeed, some SIV strains might also have evolved toward coexistence with their monkey hosts.

There is a rough parallel between the differential SAIDS susceptibility of green monkeys and macaques and the very different susceptibility to AIDS of chimpanzees and human beings. Chimpanzees are the only animals that can be experimentally infected with the HIV isolated from AIDS patients. Yet the virus does not appear to cause lethal disease in chimpanzees as it does in people. Might it be, we wondered, that chimpanzees have somehow acquired resistance to the AIDS virus? If they have, could it be because wild chimpanzees have had earlier evolutionary experience with some close relative of HIV—a relative that might, in fact, be an immediate evolutionary precursor of HIV?

R etroviruses (like other intracellular parasites) tend to coexist with their natural host species in some way that allows both to survive. In the case of some retroviruses of rodents and chickens, there has been mutual adaptation to the extent that the complete viral genome, integrated into the host genome,

is regularly inherited in all members of the host species. Such genetically inherited "endogenous" viruses have also evolved to become totally nonpathogenic. The human and simian retroviruses we are discussing, however, are "exogenous": they are transmitted horizontally, from individual to individual. It seems logical that retroviruses, like other infectious agents, may be most pathogenic when they first enter a new species. Selection for survival on the part of both the virus and the host species might then ensue.

A classic example of rapid evolution of the virus-host relation resulted from the introduction of myxoma, a lethal virus of rabbits, into Australia several decades ago. It was done deliberately, in an effort to get rid of wild rabbits that had become agricultural pests. At first the virus killed most exposed rabbits, but soon populations of rabbits emerged that were able to survive infection by the virulent myxoma virus and in the process to become immune to it. Less virulent strains of the virus also emerged; their hosts tended to survive, giving them a selective advantage over the lethal strains. Within a few years the rabbit population was restored to its original size—and the virus-host relation was completely changed.

Could the Asian macaques be analogous to the first generation of Australian rabbits, which were exposed to the myxoma virus without prior evolutionary experience and therefore died of myxomatosis? Might the African monkeys be analogous to the later, myxoma-resistant generations of rabbits? Knowing what mechanisms of immune resistance have evolved naturally in SIV-infected African monkeys, one could try to mimic such mechanisms in people exposed to HIV. The analogy between myxomatosis and SAIDS might extend to the viruses. Like the myxoma virus, HIV and SIV can mutate rapidly. Perhaps some strains of SIV, including the one that infects Asian macaques in captivity, are highly virulent and others are much less virulent. Identifying and comparing such strains could contribute to the understanding of HIV and the development of effective vaccines.

Clearly SIV is the closest known animal-virus relative of HIV. Yet it is only about 50 percent related on the basis of sequence analysis—not close enough to make it likely that SIV was an immediate precursor of HIV in people. Postulating that various HIV's and/or SIV's might exist as a spectrum of viruses in different monkey or human populations, we expanded our serological studies. Perhaps, we

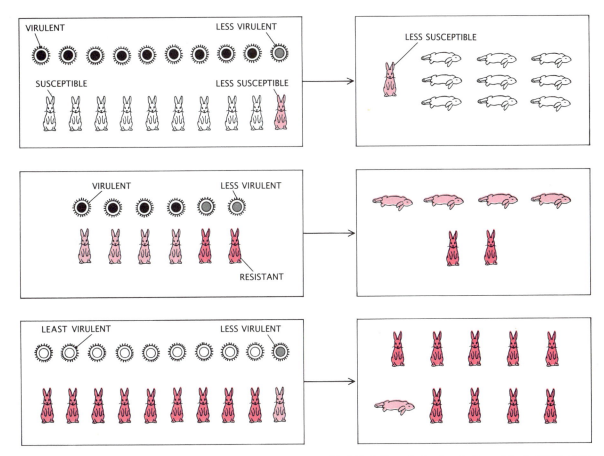

Figure 21 CASE OF THE RESISTANT RABBITS illustrates the mutual evolution of a virus and its host. Myxoma virus was introduced into Australia in an effort to get rid of wild rabbits. Virulent viruses killed most of the rabbits, but a few animals happened to be less susceptible; they survived (*right*) and multiplied. The virulent viruses eventually killed them, but a few truly resistant rabbits were spared. Meanwhile natural selection favored the evolution of avirulent virus strains (because a virus does best if its host survives). Eventually a resistant rabbit population was established, coexisting with a largely avirulent virus.

thought, one could find such a virus — an intermediate between SIV and HIV — in human beings.

To address the possibility that there might in fact be such a human virus, we examined high-risk people from diverse parts of Africa where we had earlier identified SIV-infected monkeys. We included female prostitutes, because they are at elevated risk for infection with sexually transmitted viruses; the groups that are at risk for HIV infection in industrialized countries, such as male homosexuals, intravenous drug abusers and hemophiliacs, either are rare or are difficult to identify in much of Africa.

In early 1985 we found evidence for such an SIV-related virus in Senegal in West Africa. With

our collaborators Souleymane M'Boup of the University of Dakar and Francis Barin of the University of Tours, we had tested blood-serum samples from prostitutes with antigens from both HIV and SIV. HIV-positive serums (samples known to have antibodies to HIV) from both central Africa and the U.S. were tested with the same antigens. About 10 percent of the samples from prostitutes had antibodies that reacted with both HIV and SIV. Surprisingly, the antibodies reacted much better with SIV antigens than with those of HIV, particularly with SIV's type-specific external envelope glycoprotein and envelope transmembrane protein. In contrast, the HIV-positive serums from central Africa and the

U.S. did not react very well with the SIV envelope antigens.

All in all, the reactivity of the prostitutes' antibodies to SIV antigens was indistinguishable from that of antibodies in the blood of SIV-infected macaques and African green monkeys. This clearly suggested that people in West Africa were infected with a retrovirus different from the one infecting people in central Africa, Europe and the U.S., and that the West African virus was more closely related to SIV than to HIV. Because the putative West African human virus responsible for these serological findings was clearly distinct from the AIDS virus (which in 1985 was still called HTLV-III or LAV) and would be a fourth human retrovirus, we suggested that it be designated HTLV-IV; now the original AIDS virus is called HIV-1 and the West African human virus is HIV-2.

Soon François Clavel and Luc Montagnier of the Pasteur Institute also showed that West African people were infected with a virus very similar to SIV. Their studies and ours showed that people infected with HIV-2 have antibodies entirely cross-reactive with SIV antigens; in fact, it is impossible to distinguish between SIV and HIV-2 on the basis of serological criteria.

When the genetic material of the two viruses was examined, the nucleotide sequences too were found to be closely related. All of this suggests at least that the primate and human viruses share evolutionary roots and at most that there may have been interspecies infection—that SIV-infected monkeys transmitted the virus to humans or vice versa. The sequence studies also pointed to a possibility that one of the early isolates of HIV-2 reported from our laboratory might have been from a cell culture that was contaminated with the monkey virus itself. This suspicion is based on the assumption that there cannot have been any interspecies transmission of SIV to people. It is still not possible to say with certainty how these highly related viruses came to infect their respective hosts.

Our early studies showed HIV-2 was endemic in West Africa—where there did not appear to be any clinical epidemic of AIDS. This raised new questions. Was HIV-2 minimally pathogenic in humans, as SIV seemed to be in African monkeys? HIV-2 might cause a different syndrome, one that is less severe and not as regularly lethal as HIV-1. It is also possible that AIDS cases were present in West Africa but were missed because of inadequate clinical diagnosis. Still another explanation for the seeming absence of an epidemic is the possibility that a mixture of HIV-2 strains was present in the population; differences in virulence among the strains might limit the development of AIDS to only a fraction of the infected people.

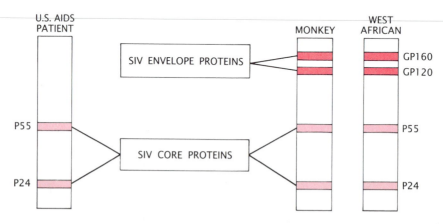

Figure 22 HIV-2 was discovered by serological testing with SIV proteins. The blood of U.S. AIDS patients had antibodies only to the core proteins, in keeping with the roughly 50 percent relation of SIV to HIV-1. As one might expect, SIV-infected monkeys had antibodies to both core and envelope proteins of SIV. People in high-risk groups in West Africa turned out also to have antibodies that reacted with both the core and the envelope proteins, indicating that they were infected by a human virus more closely related to SIV than to HIV-1. The virus is now designated HIV-2.

One could address the question of the degree of HIV-2's virulence in West African people in several ways. Clavel and Montagnier and their colleagues had isolated HIV-2 from West African AIDS patients who had been referred to Europe for treatment, suggesting that at least some strains of HIV-2 could cause AIDS. Yet the isolation from AIDS patients was not enough evidence to establish HIV-2 as a cause of AIDS. To determine whether HIV-2 strains in general were as virulent as strains of HIV-1, the epidemiology of HIV-2 had to be assessed in a number of African populations; the extent to which AIDS was associated with HIV-2 infection could help to establish the virulence of the virus.

We undertook extensive seroepidemiological studies in 14 African countries in order to determine the rates of HIV-2 and HIV-1 infection, examining more than 10,000 people in three groups: female prostitutes, patients with severe infectious diseases (such as systemic tuberculosis) that might signal an AIDS-like immune deficiency, and healthy control adults. In the controls, rates of HIV-2 infection ranged from less than 1 percent to more than 15 percent depending on location. The rates were from five to 10 times higher in female prostitutes, indicating that HIV-2, like HIV-1, is transmitted sexually. To our surprise, individuals with tuberculosis or other severe infectious diseases did not have

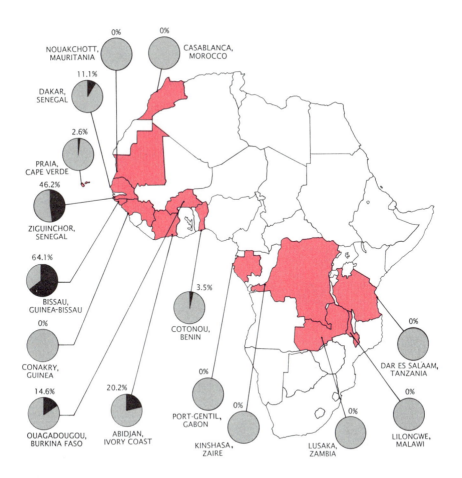

Figure 23 DISTRIBUTION OF HIV-2 in Africa was established by serological testing of female prostitutes, who constitute a high-risk group. The seroprevalence rates (the fraction of individuals who tested positive for HIV-2) are given for 15 cities in 14 countries where the test was administered. The virus appears to be limited to West Africa.

significantly higher HIV-2 rates than the controls. We found only very low rates of HIV-1 in the West African countries where HIV-2 was most prevalent. On the other hand, HIV-2 was virtually absent in the central-African countries we studied.

Prostitutes who tested positive for HIV-2 in 1985 were subsequently followed and examined carefully for abnormal clinical signs and symptoms. In contrast to prostitutes in other parts of Africa who are positive for HIV-1, they showed negligible rates of generalized lymphadenopathy (enlargement of the lymph nodes); none have shown signs or symptoms of AIDS-related complex or AIDS itself. All in all, the data suggested that West Africans infected with HIV-2 were at substantially lower risk for the development of AIDS than individuals infected with HIV-1.

Whether the difference is due to the widespread distribution of less virulent strains of HIV-2 in West Africans remains to be determined. One should also consider the possibility that HIV-2 infection of human beings is simply too new for AIDS to have developed after a long period of latent infection.

Several observations seem to argue against that possibility. One is the fact that older prostitutes have higher antibody rates than younger ones. This could simply reflect an increase in the total number of exposures to the virus with increasing age. The age effect also suggests, however, that the women who had been exposed for a long time were not being eliminated from the population pool by illness (as they would be by HIV-1 infection), and therefore that HIV-2 has been present in West African populations for a longer time but has not been very efficient at causing disease.

We also analyzed blood from patients who were in Dakar hospitals with AIDS-like illnesses, looking for evidence of infection with HIV-2 or HIV-1. Most patients had type-specific antibodies to HIV-1 rather than to HIV-2, in spite of the much lower background rates of HIV-1 infection in Dakar's population—a finding compatible with HIV-1's being more pathogenic than HIV-2. Although about 20 percent of the AIDS patients did appear to have been infected with HIV-2 rather than HIV-1, the disease seen in HIV-1-positive patients was severer

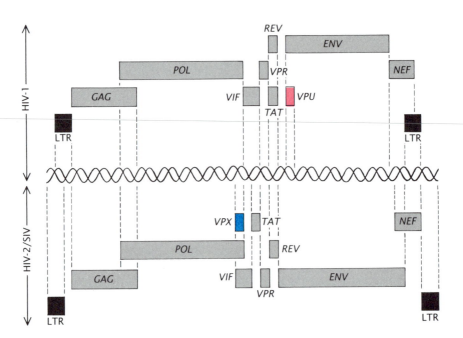

Figure 24 GENETIC ORGANIZATION of HIV-2 and SIV is compared with that of HIV-1 (*top*). The genes are arranged along the strand of proviral DNA as is shown. The *gag* gene encodes the core proteins, *env* the envelope proteins and *pol* the enzymes needed for replication. Se- quences constituting some genes overlap or are noncontiguous. The two genes that are not common to both genomes are shown in color. Knowledge of their function might help to show why HIV-1 causes lethal disease but HIV-2 may not.

and fitted a more stringent definition of AIDS. For the known human lymphotropic retroviruses, then, there appears to be a spectrum of pathogenicity. HIV-1 causes lethal disease in most infected people, whereas HTLV causes leukemia in only a few. The disease-inducing potential of HIV-2 may fall between the two.

A real difference in pathogenicity between HIV-1 and HIV-2 could be significant, and it would be important to determine its molecular basis. The two viruses infect the same populations of cells, binding to the same CD4 receptor, but there are some differences in their genetic material and therefore in their proteins. One of the most obvious is the presence in HIV-1 of the *vpu* gene, which is absent in HIV-2 (and in SIV, for that matter). Perhaps the product of this gene, a small 16-kilodalton peptide, enhances pathogenicity. Similarly, HIV-2 and SIV contain the *vpx* gene; HIV-1 does not. If this gene's 12-kilodalton product somehow slows the proliferation or spread of the virus or reduces its ability to kill cells, that too could help to explain why HIV-2 and SIV appear to be less regularly pathogenic than HIV-1.

Prostitutes from West Africa who have been infected by HIV-2 are now beginning to be exposed to HIV-1, particularly in countries such as Ivory Coast and Burkina Faso, to which HIV-1 seems to be moving from central Africa. We and others will be watching to see whether or not people previously infected by HIV-2 show decreased rates of infection with HIV-1. (Such resistance might be brought about by a number of mechanisms, including the elicitation by HIV-2 of a protective immune response to both viruses.) If individuals previously infected with HIV-2 nonetheless become infected with HIV-1, will HIV-1 then cause disease as relentlessly as it does in previously uninfected people?

Answers to these questions are likely to yield information that will help in the design of vaccines to prevent infection with HIV's. Although progress toward a vaccine against HIV-1 may have seemed to be disappointing, it appears likely that some species of monkeys, and perhaps some people, have already evolved protective mechanisms that keep certain HIV's and SIV's from causing lethal disease. Obviously one cannot simply wait for natural selection to respond (as in the case of the Australian rabbits) with the advent of more efficient immune mechanisms in people or of less virulent viruses. The challenge, then, is to understand the mechanisms that may have been involved in successful evolutionary immunoselection. Thus the origin and history of the AIDS viruses themselves may provide the very information that is critical to the prevention and control of AIDS.

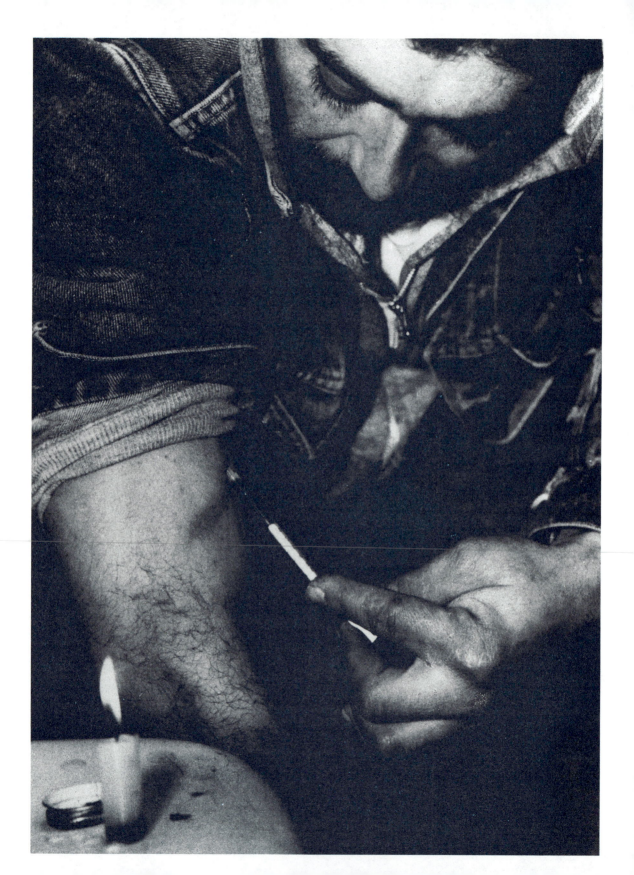

The Epidemiology of AIDS in the U.S.

In 1981 Federal officials noted that a rarely prescribed drug was being dispensed more often. It was the first sign of the AIDS epidemic. By 1992 there will probably be 365,000 cases in the U.S.

• • •

William L. Heyward and James W. Curran

Today AIDS has become a major cause of morbidity and mortality in the U.S. Indeed, it has become the leading cause of death in the country among people with hemophilia and users of illegal intravenous (IV) drugs. Moreover, nationwide morbidity and mortality rates will increase in the next few years as some of the one to 1.5 million Americans who are already infected with the human immunodeficiency virus (HIV) develop AIDS. Most of those affected in the near future will be either homosexual men or IV drug abusers, and a significant proportion of them will be blacks and Hispanics. Yet, given the fact that the virus is transmitted through sexual contact, through the traces of blood in needles and other drug paraphernalia and from mother to newborn infant, one can envision many possible chains of infection, which leave no

Figure 25 INTRAVENOUS (IV) DRUG ABUSERS share hypodermic needles and other paraphernalia that can be contaminated with blood infected with HIV. If they inject themselves with traces of the blood, they may become infected. IV drug abuse is directly or indirectly responsible for most of the HIV infections in the U.S. among heterosexual men and women as well as among infants.

segment of the U.S. population completely unaffected by the threat of AIDS.

The discovery of the epidemic, the enumeration of the varied manifestations of HIV infection and the analysis of the circumstances that made it possible for such an infection to spread have been missions assigned to epidemiology: the study of the occurrence and distribution of disease as well as its control in a given population. Epidemiologists monitor mortality and morbidity rates associated with HIV infection and AIDS; they also make predictions of likely changes in HIV infection rates in the course of time.

Most important, by carrying out studies to define the ways HIV is transmitted from person to person, epidemiologists can identify the population groups that are at greatest risk of acquiring AIDS and thereby develop strategies for the prevention and control of the disease—strategies that are independent of the development of an effective vaccine or therapy. Indeed, determining the risk factors for AIDS enabled the U.S. Public Health Service and other groups to issue recommendations for the prevention of AIDS as early as 1983, a full year before HIV was firmly identified and two years before laboratory tests to detect the presence of the virus became widely available.

To carry out all these tasks epidemiologists depend on surveillance: the gathering of high-quality, consistent and interpretable data on a disease or an infection. Surveillance data are routinely compiled from reports filed with state and local health departments that are then forwarded to the U.S. Centers for Disease Control (CDC).

It was just such a report, in June of 1981, that first alerted the CDC to AIDS. The report described how in the past eight months five cases of an extremely rare type of pneumonia caused by the protozoan *Pneumocystis carinii* had been diagnosed in the Los Angeles area. (Protozoans are a type of primitive microorganism.) This pneumonia is characteristically an opportunistic infection, occurring in people whose immune system has been profoundly impaired by cancer or by powerful immunosuppressive drugs. The disease was so uncommon that the drug given to treat it, pentamidine isethionate, was considered investigational (experimental) and could be dispensed solely by the CDC. Records at the CDC showed that between November, 1967, and December, 1979, there had been only two requests for pentamidine isethionate to treat adults who had contracted *P. carinii* pneumonia without an underlying disease. Yet in these five new cases the pneumonia had struck young homosexual men whose immune system had no apparent reason for malfunctioning.

At about the same time the CDC received reports of an increase in the incidence of a type of cancer known as Kaposi's sarcoma. The cancer had been seen only rarely in the U.S. before — predominantly in elderly men and patients receiving immunosuppressive therapy. Yet in a 30-month span 26 cases of Kaposi's sarcoma had been diagnosed among young homosexual men in New York and California. Several of these patients had also experienced *P. carinii* pneumonia and other severe opportunistic infections.

Not long afterward clinicians and epidemiologists noted an increased occurrence among homosexual men of two unexplained conditions: chronic lymphadenopathy (a condition characterized by enlarged lymph nodes) and a relatively rare malignancy called diffuse, undifferentiated non-Hodgkin's lymphoma. Once again, the only common underlying factor among the new findings and the previously reported cases of opportunistic infection and Kaposi's sarcoma was a severely impaired immune system. This collection of clinical conditions was recognized as an entirely new syndrome that became known in 1982 as acquired immunodeficiency syndrome, or AIDS.

Because the patients exhibited various common characteristics (such as age, race, city of residence and sexual orientation), it was suspected that the wide range of clinical conditions had the same underlying cause. Moreover, laboratory tests indicated that many patients with mild lymphadenopathy who did not exhibit any other signs of disease nonetheless had an abnormal immune status, suggesting there was an asymptomatic period in the patients between initial infection and the eventual development of AIDS. During this so-called latency period a person might not be ill and yet might be capable of transmitting the disease. This in turn meant that the pool of people who might be capable of transmitting the AIDS agent was significantly larger than the number of cases of AIDS reported to the CDC. AIDS was only the tip of an epidemic iceberg.

The method commonly employed by epidemiologists to determine risk factors for a particular disease is the case-control study. In this type of study people with the disease of interest (cases) are systematically compared with a similar group of people free of the disease (controls). The first national AIDS case-control study, done in 1981 among homosexual men, indicated the variable that most clearly distinguished patients with the disease from homosexual controls was the number and frequency of sexual contacts.

Another study, done in June of 1982, provided further evidence that there was an AIDS agent and that it was transmitted through sexual relations among homosexually active men. In that study data were obtained on the sexual partners of 13 of the first 19 cases of AIDS among homosexual men in the Los Angeles area. Within five years before the onset of their symptoms, nine of them had sexual contact with people who later developed Kaposi's sarcoma or *P. carinii* pneumonia. The nine were also linked to another interconnected series of 40 AIDS cases in 10 different cities by one individual who developed lymphadenopathy and was later diagnosed with Kaposi's sarcoma. Overall, investigation of these 40 cases indicated that 20 percent of the initial AIDS cases in the U.S. were linked through sexual contact —a statistical clustering that was extremely unlikely

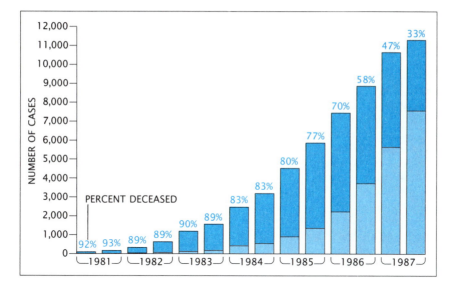

Figure 26 NUMBER OF REPORTED CASES of AIDS in the U.S. has increased each year since the disease was first recognized in 1981. The two bars for each year represent the number of cases diagnosed respectively in the first and second half of the year. The dark part of each bar corresponds to the fatality percentage among the cases. Most of the patients who were diagnosed before 1986 as having AIDS have already died.

to have occurred by chance. Still, many doubted that AIDS could be caused by a transmissible agent.

Then came the first significant evidence that other modes of transmission were possible. In 1982 AIDS cases were described among people who had been injected with blood or blood products but had no other expected risk factors. Such cases were confirmed first among people with hemophilia and then among blood-transfusion recipients as well as people who had shared hypodermic needles to inject themselves with illicit drugs.

In July, 1982, three patients with hemophilia from three different states were confirmed as having *P. carinii* pneumonia. In December of the same year an unexplained immunodeficiency with fatal *P. carinii* pneumonia was reported in a 20-month-old baby who at birth had received a blood-platelet transfusion from a man who subsequently had died of AIDS. These reports convincingly supported the hypothesis that the disease was caused by an infectious agent in the blood and perhaps in other body fluids. The reports also bolstered the evidence that the period between HIV infection and AIDS could be quite long.

During the following months several additional reports were received describing cases of AIDS in people who had received blood transfusions an average of two years before the onset of the symp-

toms. In each case at least one individual who had donated the blood for the transfusions was identified as being in a group at high risk for AIDS (such as homosexual men or IV drug abusers). These reports not only reconfirmed the transmissibility of the putative AIDS agent through blood but also emphasized the urgent need for preventing high-risk people from donating blood and for the development of laboratory tests that could detect the AIDS agent in donated blood.

In January, 1983, two well-documented AIDS cases among heterosexual partners of male IV drug abusers were reported, indicating that the AIDS agent could be clearly transmitted to an infected man's heterosexual partners as well as his homosexual ones. Later that year AIDS cases were first recognized in people from central Africa and Haiti who had no history of homosexuality or IV drug abuse. It became increasingly evident that AIDS was a sexually transmitted disease and that the most important risk factor was the relative number of different sex partners—not necessarily sexual preference. It was also evident that the extent of homosexual transmission of AIDS in relation to its heterosexual transmission varied from country to country.

Because the disease appeared to be transmitted through the exchange of blood or by sexual contact, most investigators were convinced by late 1982 that the cause of AIDS was an infectious agent (most likely a virus) and not the result of exposure to toxic substances or other environmental or genetic factors. The infection hypothesis was finally confirmed when HIV was isolated by Luc Montagnier and his colleagues at the Pasteur Institute in Paris and by Robert C. Gallo and his colleagues at the National Cancer Institute.

Soon after the discovery of the AIDS agent a laboratory test was developed to detect antibodies to HIV in the blood. A positive result in a test of a person's blood sample was a reliable sign that the person was infected with the virus. Such a serological test made it possible to detect HIV infection in people who showed no clinical symptoms, and to confirm clinical diagnoses of AIDS and other HIV-related conditions. It also made it possible to measure directly the prevalence of HIV infection (the number of infected people in a given population at a given time) and its incidence (the number of new infections occurring within a defined period in a specific population). Most important, perhaps, was the fact that the national supply of donated blood could now be screened, so that additional cases of AIDS due to blood transfusions and contaminated blood products could be avoided.

Serological studies among high-risk groups soon confirmed what had originally been suspected: the AIDS cases recorded so far constituted just a fraction of the total number of people infected with HIV. These studies made possible a clearer definition of the disease's modes of transmission, the factors affecting the risk of infection and the specific population groups that should be targeted for prevention and control measures. The serological test also clarified the clinical spectrum of the disease and enabled the CDC to formulate a more precise "case definition" of AIDS that made the diagnosis and reporting of AIDS cases more consistent nationwide.

AIDS cases (along with cases of other diseases or health conditions) are reported to state or local health agencies. Currently all 50 states, the District of Columbia and Puerto Rico require that all such reports be passed along, without identifying the individual patients, to the CDC. The primary sources of surveillance data on AIDS therefore include hospitals, clinics, physicians and medical-record systems (which handle such matters as death certificates, tumor registries, communicable-disease reports and hospital-discharge summaries).

The main concern about any surveillance system is the completeness of the reporting. One way to measure this is to compare reports from various surveillance sources. Recent studies in five major cities showed that at least 90 percent of the diagnoses meeting the AIDS case definition were in fact reported. This rate of reporting is extraordinarily high compared with that for most other diseases, for which only between 10 and 25 percent of the cases are typically reported.

As of July 4, 1988, a total of 66,464 adults and children have been reported as AIDS cases to the CDC. Of these, 37,535 — more than half — have died, including more than 80 percent of the patients diagnosed before 1985. Since 1981, when reporting of AIDS cases began, 63 percent of the victims of the disease in the U.S. have been homosexual or bisexual men without a history of IV drug abuse, 7 percent were homosexual or bisexual men with a history of IV drug abuse and 19 percent were heterosexual men and women who were IV drug abusers. In addition almost 3 percent of all the recorded AIDS cases were associated with transfusions of contaminated blood, nearly all of which had been received before 1985 (when serological screening of blood donors was instituted); roughly 1 percent of the adults who contracted AIDS were hemophiliacs. The means by which the HIV infection was acquired was undetermined in only 3 percent of adults with AIDS, generally because of incomplete information on the frequency of their sexual contacts, among other factors .

Of the 2,702 AIDS cases attributed to heterosexual transmission (representing 4 percent of the total), 1,643 (367 men and 1,276 women) had a history of sexual contact with a person documented as having been infected with HIV or with a person in another risk category. Another 1,059 were born in countries where heterosexual contact is the major mode of transmission. The 1:3.5 ratio of male to female cases of heterosexually transmitted AIDS in the U.S. is probably due to a larger pool of men infected by other means, such as IV drug abuse and homosexual contact. It is also possible that male-to-female transmission is more efficient than female-to-male transmission.

The members of the fastest growing group of reported AIDS patients are not adults; they are children. In the past 12 months 502 cases of AIDS have been reported in children under 13 years old — a 114 percent increase over the previous 12-month period. A total of 1,054 such pediatric cases have

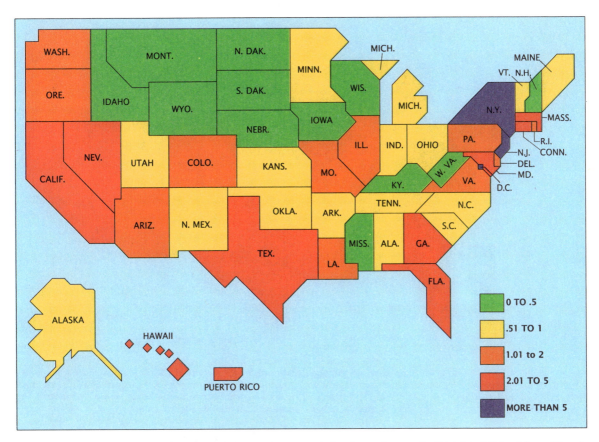

Figure 27 GEOGRAPHIC DISTRIBUTION of AIDS shows that the Northeast has been most affected. The map displays the cumulative reported cases of AIDS per 10,000 population for each state, the District of Columbia and Puerto Rico as of March 28, 1988.

now been recorded. In 78 percent of them the HIV infection was acquired perinatally (before, during or soon after birth). Most of these pediatric cases can be traced to IV drug use by the child's mother or her sexual partner. In 19 percent of all pediatric cases the source of HIV infection was either a blood transfusion or treatment for hemophilia.

In the U.S. 59 percent of the reported AIDS cases among adults and 23 percent of the cases among children have been white; blacks have accounted for 26 percent of adult cases and 53 percent of pediatric cases, and Hispanics for 14 percent of adult and 23 percent of pediatric cases. Such figures are in striking contrast to the respective percentages of blacks (11.6 percent) and Hispanics (6.5 percent) in the general U.S. population.

The disproportionate percentage of AIDS cases among blacks and Hispanics largely reflects higher reported rates of AIDS in black and Hispanic IV drug abusers, their sex partners and their infants. Because of the high concentration of IV drug abuse in the Northeast, the risk of contracting AIDS is between two and 10 times higher for blacks and Hispanics living in that region than it is elsewhere in the country. Rates for transfusion-associated AIDS do not differ significantly when they are divided by race or ethnicity for adult cases, although the rates are significantly higher for black infants—perhaps owing to a greater need for transfusions to manage low birth weight in black newborns.

The human immunodeficiency virus is transmitted primarily through sexual contact, exposure to blood and blood products and from mother to child during the perinatal period. In the U.S. most sexual transmission of HIV has been among homo-

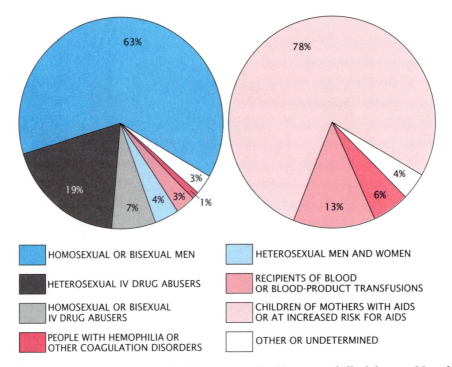

HOMOSEXUAL OR BISEXUAL MEN

HETEROSEXUAL IV DRUG ABUSERS

HOMOSEXUAL OR BISEXUAL
IV DRUG ABUSERS

PEOPLE WITH HEMOPHILIA OR
OTHER COAGULATION DISORDERS

HETEROSEXUAL MEN AND WOMEN

RECIPIENTS OF BLOOD
OR BLOOD-PRODUCT TRANSFUSIONS

CHILDREN OF MOTHERS WITH AIDS
OR AT INCREASED RISK FOR AIDS

OTHER OR UNDETERMINED

Figure 28 POPULATION GROUPS accounting for the adult (*left*) and pediatric (*right*) cases of AIDS as of July 4, 1988, are indicated by these pie charts. As can be seen, homosexual or bisexual men and IV drug abusers together account for 89 percent of all adult cases. More than three-fourths of the children with AIDS acquired the disease from a mother who either had AIDS or was a member of the group at increased risk for AIDS.

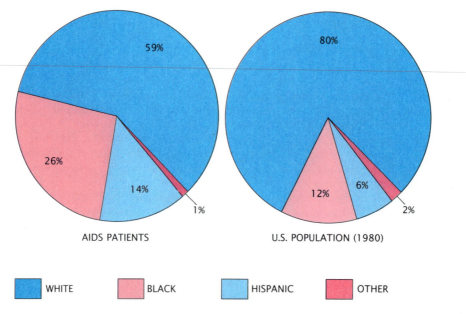

AIDS PATIENTS

U.S. POPULATION (1980)

WHITE   BLACK   HISPANIC   OTHER

Figure 29 RACIAL AND ETHNIC CLASSIFICATION of the adult AIDS cases shows a disproportionate fraction of them are among blacks and Hispanics. The figures reflect the higher reported rates of AIDS in black and Hispanic IV drug abusers and their sex partners.

sexual men. The risk of infection in these men increases with the number of sexual partners and the frequency with which they are the receptive partner in anal intercourse. The insertive partner in anal intercourse, however, has also been known to become infected with HIV, and one report has described infection in the receptive partner in orogenital intercourse. The relative efficiency of transmission for different types of sexual practices is difficult to determine precisely, because most homosexual men in studies have engaged in multiple practices. As in the case of other sexually transmitted diseases, the frequency of female-to-female transmission is very low, although at least one such case (involving the tearing of skin and mucous membranes) has been reported.

Syphilis and genital herpes, as well as other causes of genital or anal ulcers, have been associated with HIV infection in homosexual men in the U.S. and in heterosexuals in central Africa. It is supposed that the damage done to the genital skin and mucous membranes by these infections may facilitate HIV acquisition or transmission. If sexually transmitted genital-ulcer diseases increase the transmission rate of HIV, then populations with high rates of venereal disease are likely to be at increased risk for HIV infection. Prevention and prompt treatment of sexually transmitted infections could potentially slow the spread of HIV among sexually active men and women.

Although there have been many documented cases of male-to-female as well as female-to-male sexual transmission of HIV, the study populations have been too small to allow a comparison of the relative efficiencies of transmission in the two directions. Most heterosexual transmission of HIV occurs during vaginal intercourse, but two small studies have suggested that anal intercourse increases the risk of infection in women. The cumulative rate of infection has been reported to be significantly higher among the female partners of infected male IV drug abusers and men from Haiti or countries in central Africa than it is among female partners of infected men in other risk groups (including bisexual men, hemophiliacs and transfusion recipients). Among heterosexual couples in which one partner (the "index" case) is infected with HIV, from 10 to 70 percent of the other partners have become infected through sexual intercourse.

This variability in infection rate is not fully explained by the frequency of sexual contact; it may have something to do with how long the index case

has been infected. Recently it has been shown that people with AIDS or symptomatic HIV infection are more likely to transmit HIV infection than those who are asymptomatic or at an earlier stage of infection. Nevertheless, partners in some such couples have managed to remain uninfected, in spite of the fact that the couples had long-standing sexual relations and took no precautions against infection.

These findings suggest that, in addition to behavioral factors, biological factors often contribute to HIV transmission. It also appears that some infected individuals may be more efficient transmitters of HIV than others and that a person's infectiousness may vary with time.

Transfusion of a single unit of HIV-contaminated blood is very likely to result in infection; between 89 and 100 percent of recipients of contaminated blood are reported to become infected. Fortunately transfusion of HIV-infected blood in the U.S. is now rare, since high-risk people are discouraged from donating blood and all donated blood is screened for HIV antibodies. Because the sharing of needles and other drug-related paraphernalia also provides a way for contaminated blood to be injected into the body (in amounts substantially smaller than those involved in transfusions), that activity can result in HIV transmission as well. Indeed, in the U.S. IV drug abuse is now the major source of HIV transmission in heterosexual men and women and, consequently, of perinatal transmission as well.

The possibility that one can become infected with HIV if contaminated blood penetrates the skin or mucous membranes also represents a small but definite occupational risk for health-care workers. In a national collaborative study done by the CDC, four of 870 health-care workers who had accidentally punctured their skin with needles contaminated with the blood of HIV-infected people developed HIV infection, but none of the 104 workers whose mucous membranes or skin had been exposed to blood became infected. In another study of health-care workers at the National Institutes of Health, no HIV infections occurred among 103 workers with needle-stick injuries, nor were there any HIV infections among 691 workers who had a total of more than 2,000 reported skin and mucous-membrane exposures to blood or body fluids of AIDS patients. These studies are consistent with other data indicating that the occupational risk of acquiring HIV infection in health-care settings is low and is most

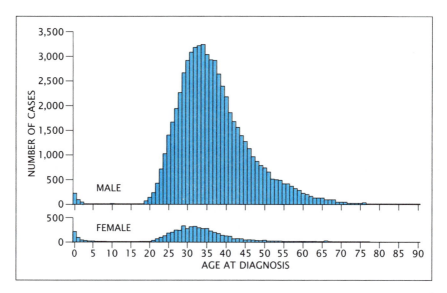

Figure 30 AGE DISTRIBUTIONS for male and female AIDS patients in the U.S. indicate that most patients are males between the ages of 25 and 45. The distinct peaks at the left of the distributions represent the small but increasing number of pediatric AIDS cases.

often associated with percutaneous inoculation of blood from an infected patient.

HIV is also transmitted from an infected mother to her newborn child, but the extent of transmission that takes place respectively during pregnancy, at birth or soon afterward is as yet unknown. Detection of HIV in fetal tissues supports the hypothesis that infection occurs in utero, and case reports of women who became infected with HIV immediately after giving birth, and subsequently infected their infants, suggest that the virus may be transmitted through breast-feeding.

Studies of such perinatal transmission are greatly complicated by the lack of a reliable diagnostic test to determine HIV infection in newborns. As is the case with other infections, infants born to HIV-infected mothers have maternally derived HIV antibodies circulating in their blood—regardless of whether or not they have been infected. The maternal HIV antibodies may persist for as long as 12 months and cannot be distinguished from antibodies that may be present in an infant infected with HIV. Other tests are under development for identifying HIV infection in these newborns. Currently all infants born to infected mothers must be followed closely for at least 12 months to see whether there is any clinical or laboratory evidence of HIV infection or AIDS.

There has been considerable concern that in rare circumstances other types of transmission might occur—particularly through casual contact with HIV-infected people or by way of insect vectors. Although HIV has been recovered from the saliva of infected individuals, the virus concentration is much lower in saliva than it is in blood. In a CDC study not one of 48 health-care workers became infected after skin or mucous-membrane exposure to the saliva of HIV-infected people.

To evaluate the risk of HIV transmission through other casual contacts, several prospective studies (which are carried out over several years) have been done of the families of infected adults and children. In spite of tens of thousands of days of household contact with infected individuals, not one of more than 400 family members has been infected with HIV—except for sexual partners of the infected person and children born to infected mothers. In these studies the documented risk of household transmission was zero, and therefore the actual risk must be extremely low, even in crowded households. The risk of transmission in other social settings, such as schools and offices, is presumably even lower than in household settings.

Epidemiological studies in the U.S. and other countries throughout the world show no patterns of HIV infection consistent with transmission by insect

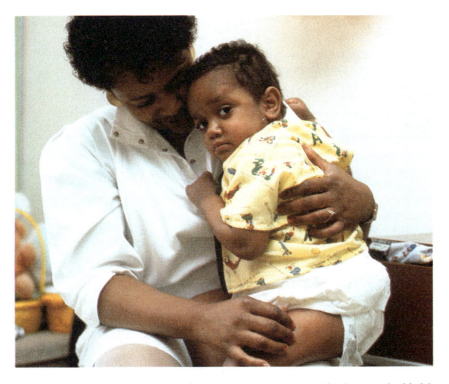

Figure 31 FIVE-YEAR-OLD AIDS PATIENT is one of the increasing number of children who have become infected with HIV perinatally: before, during or soon after birth. Reports of such pediatric cases doubled in number in a recent 12-month period.

vectors. If HIV were transmitted by insect vectors, additional cases of infection would be seen in people who share environments with infected individuals. Such evidence is lacking, in spite of extensive surveillance efforts. In addition there is a relative absence of HIV infection in African preadolescent children—another fact that argues against insects as an important mode of transmission. Although HIV can survive from several hours up to several days in insects artificially fed blood with high concentrations of the virus, there is no evidence that HIV actually grows in insects. Such a biological event is important in most viral diseases transmitted by insects.

To be sure, the existence of other unrecognized modes of HIV transmission can never be entirely excluded, but if they do exist, they appear to be extremely rare.

Mathematical models have been developed to predict the future course of HIV infection and AIDS in the U.S. These models, which are useful for planning public-health programs, take into account the natural history of HIV infection and make certain assumptions about the size of the population groups at risk, diagnostic and reporting practices and the incidence of infection. The projections must also adjust for the prolonged latency period of AIDS. (It is now estimated that about half of the people infected with HIV will develop AIDS in 10 years.)

The Public Health Service estimates that currently a total of between one and 1.5 million people in the U.S. are infected with HIV. Yet since the epidemic of HIV infection in the U.S. is actually a composite of many partially overlapping epidemics, each with its own rate of spread, there must be estimates of incidence in each of the groups at risk for AIDS in order to predict accurately the future course of the overall epidemic. Unfortunately the accurate data necessary for detailed estimates of the incidence and prevalence of HIV infection in most specific groups and geographic areas are not currently available. Obtaining the data is therefore a priority of the Public Health Service as well as state and local public-health departments.

At least two methods have been utilized to forecast short-term future trends of AIDS in the U.S. One method, employed by W. Meade Morgan and John Karon of the CDC, involves fitting a curve to the cases of AIDS reported in the past and extrapolating it into the future. Another approach, called the back-calculation method, is used by Ronald Brookmeyer and his collaborators at the Johns Hopkins University School of Hygiene and Public Health. This method makes use of current AIDS incidence data and estimates of the latency-period distribution to predict the future trend of AIDS incidence.

For both models projections of current HIV prevalence and trends in AIDS incidence over the next few years are nearly the same. The extrapolation model predicts that about 39,000 cases of AIDS will have been diagnosed during 1988, and that the annual-incidence figure will increase to 60,000 in 1990. It also projects that the cumulative case count will reach 365,000 by the end of 1992. Although the uncertainty associated with these projections increases the further into the future one goes, in the two years that have passed since the initial projection was made more than 95 percent of the total projected cases have in fact been reported to the CDC.

Since the latency period may be as long as several years, the incidence of reported AIDS cases will continue to increase for many years after the incidence of HIV infection has stabilized or begun to decline. Although current data are not yet sufficient to determine whether the overall annual incidence of HIV infection has in fact stabilized, the data are encouraging for homosexual men, transfusion recipients and people with hemophilia.

Extensive studies of homosexual men followed over a period of several years consistently show lower rates of incidence for HIV infection between 1985 and 1987 compared with the early 1980's. This decrease can be at least partially attributed to marked changes in sexual behavior in homosexual men, as is demonstrated in several other studies. Perhaps as a result of these changes, there has also been a marked decline in reported syphilis and gonorrhea cases in the group.

In spite of these downward trends, the recent decrease in incidence rates for homosexual men is not uniform and certainly the risk of HIV infection for homosexual men remains high. In contrast, since the screening of blood and blood products for HIV antibodies was instituted, the incidence of HIV infection among people with hemophilia and among blood-transfusion recipients has dropped precipitously.

More than 30 months of serological testing of applicants for military service has shown stable or declining HIV-infection rates among the applicants,

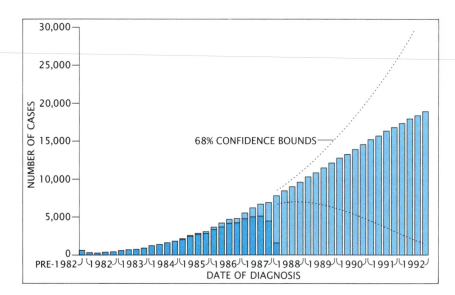

Figure 32 QUARTERLY INCIDENCE of AIDS in the U.S. is projected through 1992 by extrapolating pre-1987 trends. Actual cases reported to the Centers for Disease Control in Atlanta through March 31, 1988 (*color*), account for about 90 percent of the total projected.

both as a group and when they are analyzed by age, sex, race, ethnicity or geographic region. These results suggest that people likely to be infected are selectively avoiding enlisting, making the data difficult to interpret. Nevertheless, these data do not suggest an explosive rise in infection in the population from which military applicants are drawn.

Incidence rates are measured directly among groups in which the same people are tested more than once. Accurate determination of the incidence of HIV infection in the U.S. will remain a challenge, since people who have just become infected seldom seek medical care and it is hard to sample truly representative populations. As a consequence, trends in prevalence among groups that are available for HIV testing must be used to estimate overall trends of HIV infection.

The strategy for controlling HIV infection and AIDS in the U.S. involves educating and counseling people on how to avoid behavior that results in the transmission of HIV. Counseling people found to be infected with HIV involves not only advising them and their sexual partners on how to avoid HIV transmission but also providing them with medical care, social services and perhaps treatment for drug addiction. Indeed, the treatment and prevention of IV drug abuse, so that the sharing of HIV-contaminated needles and other drug-related equipment is reduced, will be a crucial step in preventing HIV transmission in the U.S.

Many gaps remain in our understanding of the dynamics of HIV infection in the U.S. At the state and local level the highest priorities should be to understand better the precise populations at risk for HIV infection and to apply this information in directing and monitoring specific prevention programs. These efforts in both investigative and applied epidemiology will have to be expanded rapidly and continued for the foreseeable future in order to limit the further spread of HIV in the U.S.

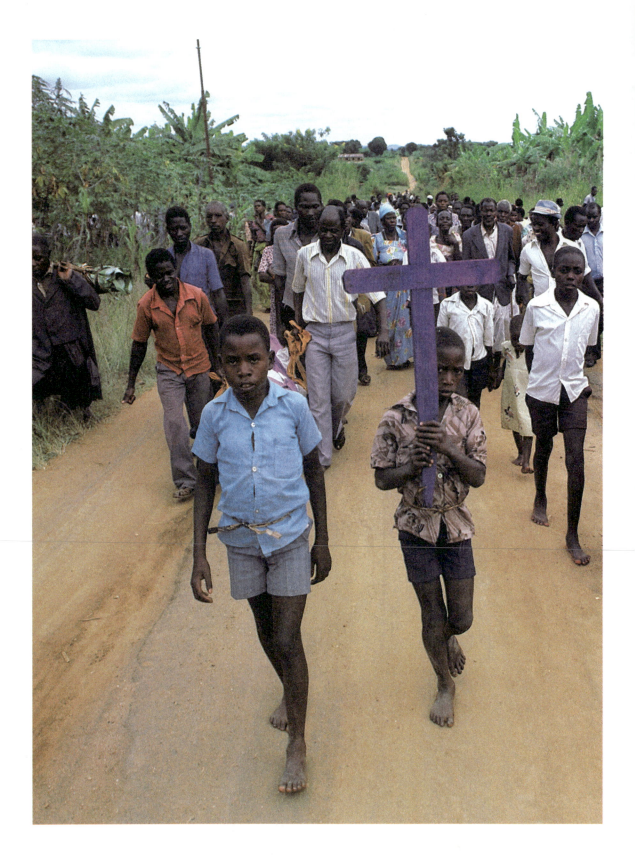

The International Epidemiology of AIDS

Reports to the World Health Organization suggest that at least five million people worldwide are infected by the AIDS virus and a million new cases of AIDS are likely within the next five years.

. . .

Jonathan M. Mann, James Chin, Peter Piot and Thomas Quinn

Ever since the AIDS pandemic was initially recognized in 1981 it has been met by denial and a gross underestimation of its potential magnitude. The pandemic is still in its early stages and its ultimate dimensions are difficult to gauge, but by now it is apparent that AIDS is an unprecedented threat to global health. From our current knowledge of the disease, we estimate that over 250,000 cases of AIDS have already occurred, that between five and 10 million people worldwide are infected with the AIDS virus and that within the next five years about one million new AIDS cases can be expected. In short, the global situation will get much worse before it can be brought under control.

This grim prognosis is based on numerous epidemiological studies that have clarified the current distribution patterns of human immunodeficiency

Figure 33 FUNERALS FOR AIDS VICTIMS are daily occurrences in Kyotera, a town in Uganda from which most of the merchants have fled and where most of the children are now orphans. HIV, which causes AIDS, infects as many as 15 or 20 percent of certain segments of the adult urban population of Uganda, as well as that of the Congo, Rwanda, Tanzania, Zaire and Zambia.

virus (HIV), which causes AIDS, and its various modes of transmission. Worldwide surveillance of AIDS, from which the global distribution pattern is determined, is coordinated by the Global Program on AIDS (GPA) at the World Health Organization (WHO) in Geneva. Reports to Geneva are received from the WHO's regional offices and individual countries' ministries of health. The accuracy and completeness of AIDS reporting vary in different areas of the world. In the U.S., validation studies by the Centers for Disease Control in Atlanta have indicated that from 80 to 90 percent of diagnosed cases are in fact reported. In most developed countries, it is thought that the majority of diagnosed cases are reported to national health authorities. On the other hand, it is thought that in most developing countries the majority of AIDS cases to date have not been reported to the WHO because of significant underrecognition, underdiagnosis and underreporting.

The thousands of AIDS cases now being reported every year are due to HIV infections that began spreading silently and extensively in the 1970's, before the disease was even recognized and before

HIV was isolated. Although blood stored as early as 1959 in Zaire has been found to contain antibodies against the AIDS virus, the actual origin of HIV is still not known with any certainty; this ignorance was underscored when in 1987 the World Health Assembly stated that HIV is a "naturally occurring retrovirus of undetermined geographic origin." In 1985 a related virus was discovered in West Africa. The original virus and the newer one are now referred to as HIV-1 and HIV-2 respectively. Although preliminary observations suggest that HIV-2 infections may be less pathogenic than those of HIV-1, the natural history of HIV-2 has not been fully established and for the purposes of this article the two viruses are assumed to have similar effects.

By now a clear picture of how HIV is transmitted has emerged. Studies have consistently shown that the virus is transmitted by sexual intercourse (vaginal or anal), by the injection or administration of infected blood or from an infected mother to her infant. There is no evidence to support transmission by food or water, by biting insects or by coughing or sneezing. Most important, there is no evidence for casual transmission between people in schools, in the workplace or other such social settings. Individual reports and rumors to the contrary should not be allowed to distort the basic facts about transmission, because an understanding of how HIV is spread and not spread is central to the development of appropriate and effective control measures.

After infection a person may remain symptom-free for years. An unknown proportion of infected people do experience an early, brief, mononucleosis-like illness with fever, malaise and possibly a skin rash. Such symptoms, when they are present, develop at about the time antibodies produced by the body against HIV can first be detected. This usually occurs between two weeks and three months after infection, rarely later. From that point on an average of eight or nine years may pass before AIDS is fully developed. The fatality rate for AIDS, once it has developed, is very high; it may reach 100 percent. The interval between diagnosis of AIDS to death varies greatly: in developed countries about 50 percent of the patients die within 18 months of diagnosis, and 80 percent die within 36 months. Survival times appear to be shorter in Africa and Haiti, but this may be due to later diagnosis and limited medical facilities. To date no study has found any resistance to HIV among any race group.

Since HIV infection precedes the development of AIDS by at least several years, to get a good picture of the disease's current distribution one cannot rely solely on reported AIDS cases; it is also necessary to collect data on the number or proportion of people who are infected with HIV. Such "seroprevalence data" indicate by the presence in the blood of antibodies against HIV, that a person has been infected by the virus. From analyses of both AIDS reports and seroprevalence data three broad, and yet distinct, patterns of AIDS have been recognized.

Pattern I is typical of industrialized countries with large numbers of reported AIDS cases. These countries include the U.S., Mexico and Canada, many Western European countries, Australia, New Zealand and parts of Latin America. Some regions of South Africa also exhibit pattern-I behavior, though these areas are not industrialized. In pattern-I countries HIV probably began to spread extensively in the late 1970's. Most cases occur among homosexual or bisexual males and urban intravenous (IV) drug users. Heterosexual transmission is responsible for only a small percentage of cases but is increasing. There was transmission due to the transfusion of some blood and blood products between the late 1970's and 1985, but that route has now been practically eliminated by convincing people in high-risk groups not to donate blood and by routine, effective testing of blood donors for antibodies against HIV. Unsterile needles, except those used by IV drug users, are not a significant factor in HIV transmission in pattern-I countries.

In pattern-I areas the male-to-female sex ratio of reported AIDS cases ranges from 10 to one to 15 to one. Because relatively few women are infected in these areas, to date perinatal transmission (transmission from mother to infant) is not common. In the overall population of pattern-I countries, infection by HIV is estimated (on the basis of seroprevalence data) to be less than 1 percent, but it has been measured at more than 50 percent in some groups practicing high-risk behavior: men with multiple male sex partners and IV drug users who share unsterile needles or syringes.

Pattern II is presently observed in some areas of central, eastern and southern Africa and increasingly in certain Latin American countries, particularly those of the Caribbean. Like pattern-I areas, pattern-II areas probably saw the extensive spread of HIV beginning in the late 1970's. In contrast to pattern-I areas, however, most cases in pattern-II areas occur among heterosexuals and the ratio of infected males to females is approximately one to one. Transmission through homosexual activity or IV drug use is either absent or at a very low level, but because many women are infected, perinatal transmission is common.

Pattern III prevails in areas of Eastern Europe, North Africa, the Middle East, Asia and most of the Pacific (excluding Australia and New Zealand). In pattern-III countries, HIV was probably introduced in the early to mid-1980's, and only a small number of AIDS cases has so far been reported. These have generally occurred in people who have traveled to pattern-I or pattern-II areas and who have had sexual contact with individuals from such areas. Indigenous homosexual, heterosexual and IV-drug-use transmission have only recently been documented. Some cases have been caused by imported blood or blood products and, in a few pattern-III countries, they account for the largest percentage of reported AIDS cases to date.

With these infection and disease patterns as a guide, we shall now examine the geographical distribution of AIDS in more detail, concentrating on the epidemiology outside North America (see Chapter

4, "The Epidemiology of AIDS in the U.S.," by William L. Heyward and James W. Curran).

The continent hardest hit by the AIDS pandemic is Africa where all three infection patterns can be found. Patterns I and II are seen in South Africa. Pattern III prevails in North Africa, including most countries in the Sahel region. In sub-Saharan Africa, below the Sahel, pattern II prevails in the large urban areas of central, eastern and southern Africa. In West African countries, where pattern II is also found, HIV-2 infections are much more common than HIV-1 infections. AIDS cases are being increasingly detected in West Africa; whether HIV-2 will ultimately prove to be as pathogenic as HIV-1 remains an open question and is the subject of intense epidemiological and clinical research.

AIDS has become one of the major health problems that confront the countries of central and eastern Africa in particular. In many of the urban centers of the Congo, Rwanda, Tanzania, Uganda, Zaire and Zambia from 5 to 20 percent of the sexually active age-group has already been infected with HIV. Rates of infection among some prostitute

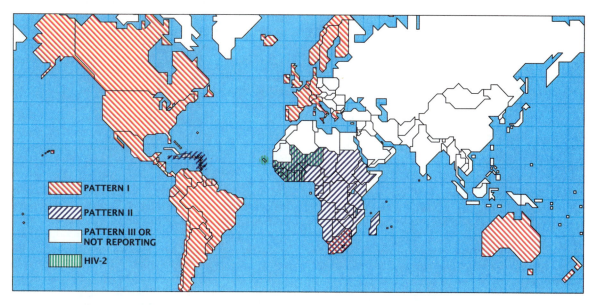

Figure 34 THREE INFECTION PATTERNS of the AIDS virus are apparent worldwide. Pattern I is found in North and South America, Western Europe, Scandinavia, Australia and New Zealand. In these areas about 90 percent of the cases are homosexual males or users of intravenous drugs. Pattern II is found in Africa, the Caribbean and some areas of South America; the primary mode of transmission in these regions is heterosexual sex and the number of infected females and males is approximately equal. Pattern III is typical of Eastern Europe, North Africa, the Middle East, Asia and the Pacific (excluding Australia and New Zealand); there are relatively few cases and most of them have had contact with pattern-I or pattern-II countries.

groups range from 27 percent in Kinshasa, Zaire, to 66 percent in Nairobi, Kenya, and 88 percent in Butare, Rwanda. Close to half of all patients in the medical wards of hospitals in those cities are currently infected with HIV. So are from 10 to 25 percent of the women of childbearing age, and that will mean an increase in child mortality by at least 25 percent; the gains achieved with difficulty by child-survival programs over the past two decades may be nullified. By the early 1990's the total adult mortality rate in these urban areas will have been doubled or tripled by AIDS.

As bleak as this picture is, the situation could become even worse if the AIDS epidemic spreads significantly from urban areas, where it is now focused and which contain only from 10 to 20 percent of the population, to the rural areas where most people live. The cumulative total of AIDS cases in Africa by mid-1988 was estimated at more than 100,000, and health-care systems in developing African countries are often unable to cope with the current patient load. How these health-care systems will be able to manage the additional 400,000 cases projected within the next five years in urban areas is a problem seeking solutions; it will be a severe challenge not only to the countries directly affected but to external assistance groups.

In pattern-I countries, for example the U.S., HIV infection is found overwhelmingly among male homosexuals and IV drug users. In contrast, the major characteristic of the pattern-II infection in most of sub-Saharan Africa is its prevalence among heterosexuals. What accounts for the difference?

Widespread IV drug use, which would lead to increased heterosexual transmission, is not a significant problem in sub-Saharan Africa; although homosexuality exists worldwide, it has not been documented to any appreciable extent among AIDS cases or HIV-infected people in sub-Saharan Africa. Many epidemiological studies have shown that transfusion of HIV-infected blood can account for only a small fraction of the infections in sub-Saharan Africa. The use of unsterile needles or other skin-piercing instruments within the health-care system or as part of traditional healing practices also accounts for only a small portion of HIV infections in these areas. Ritual surgical removal of the clitoris in females has been postulated to be an important factor in the spread of HIV. The areas where such so-called circumcisions are still carried out, however, do not in general coincide with the areas where HIV or AIDS is currently most prevalent.

Genetic differences between pattern-I and pattern-II populations have also been proposed by several Indian and Caribbean investigators to explain the level and extent of heterosexual transmission in Africa. Yet no genetic basis has been identified among race groups for either increased susceptibility to infection or the capacity to disseminate HIV. Neither have virological studies so far revealed any difference among any strains of HIV that would result in increased infectious capability and hence the large number of infections among Africans.

Given that the above factors do not appear to contribute significantly to the spread of AIDS in Africa, one returns to what is well established: the likelihood of sexual transmission of HIV appears to be governed by the probability of exposure to an infected partner as well as the specific sexual acts performed with that partner. Although systematic studies of sexual behavior in sub-Saharan Africa are not yet available, investigators have generally reported a greater number of sexual partners and/or contacts with female prostitutes among African males who have AIDS than among control groups. High rates of partner exchange, or the frequent exposure to a relatively small number of prostitutes of many men who then return to their spouses, could contribute to the epidemiological pattern of HIV infection in these areas. Among sexual practices, available studies strongly suggest that vaginal intercourse is the dominant behavior in sub-Saharan Africa, reinforcing the supposition that frequency of sexual contact is the primary factor governing the transmission of HIV there.

Certain aggravating factors may help to explain possible differences in susceptibility to HIV infection. For example, individuals whose immune system has been activated by chronic infections might be more easily infected on exposure to HIV. There is also increasing evidence that the presence of other sexually transmitted diseases increases the risk of HIV infection. Studies in Africa indicate that such diseases (in particular those characterized by genital ulceration, such as chancroid and syphilis) may increase susceptibility to infection on exposure to a partner carrying HIV or may increase the infectivity of a person carrying HIV. Studies in the U.S. show that HIV infection is positively correlated with the presence of genital or anal lesions in homosexual men. Moreover, the higher prevalence of sexually transmitted diseases, including chancroid and syphilis, in tropical Africa compared with general populations in Europe is consistent with the hypothesis

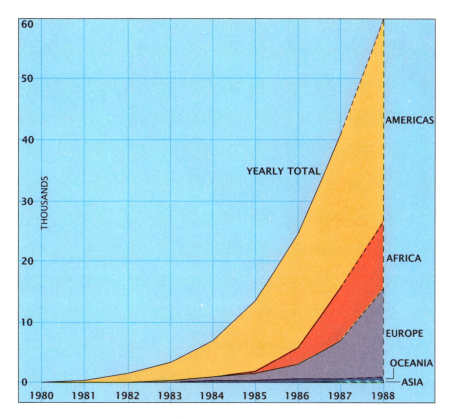

Figure 35 NUMBER OF AIDS CASES reported to the World Health Organization (WHO) in each year from 1980 to 1988 is shown. The 1988 data, indicated by dashed lines, are projections. The Americas dominate the number of reported cases in part because of high reporting efficiency, which perhaps approaches 90 percent. The total-cases curve exhibits nearly exponential growth, with a doubling time of slightly over a year. This striking rate of increase is due not only to an actual increase in the number of AIDS cases but also to improved surveillance. The cumulative total as of August 1, 1988, was 108,176. Underreporting is still a problem in many parts of the world, however, and the WHO estimates that the true total was actually close to 250,000.

that such diseases aggravate the spread of AIDS in Africa.

Turning from Africa to Asia and the Pacific, one finds a less grim situation. In Oceania, as of June 1, 1988, four countries have reported a total of 892 cases of AIDS, all but two of which were reported by Australia (813) and New Zealand (77). These two countries exhibit the pattern-I infection characteristic of the U.S. Other countries in Asia and the Pacific have generally low levels of HIV infection and few AIDS patients. In these areas HIV infection and AIDS have been detected mainly in people who have visited a pattern-I or pattern-II country or have had sexual or needle-sharing contact with people from such countries.

In China and Japan the largest number of docu- mented HIV infections are among those people to whom imported blood or blood products were administered before 1986. Still, in absolute and relative terms the number is very small. Among blood donors in Hong Kong and Singapore, only about one person in from 50,000 to 80,000 have been found HIV seropositive, that is, to have antibodies against HIV. In female prostitute populations, the HIV infection rate has been found to be either zero or at most about one per 1,000. Small pockets of relatively high infection rates, however, have been found among some prostitute groups in the Philippines, where up to .5 percent may be infected, and in India, where up to 6 percent may be infected.

In Asian and Pacific countries HIV infections do not appear to be spreading rapidly among the general heterosexual population, but intensive surveil-

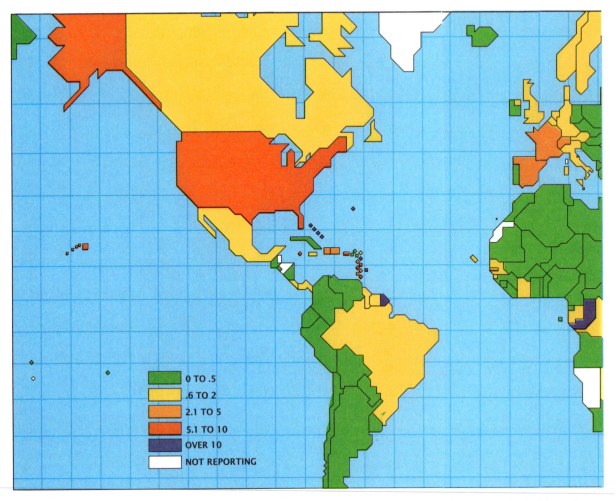

Figure 36 REPORTED AIDS CASES per 100,000 of population are mapped for 1987. Displaying the case rate rather than absolute numbers has the advantage of showing approximately what proportion of the population has AIDS. Such data do, however, tend to overstate the incidence in small countries with good AIDS surveillance; the incidence tends to be understated for countries that do not report most cases to the WHO.

lance of prostitutes and patients with sexually transmitted diseases is being undertaken to monitor this situation closely. Of great public concern in Thailand was the documentation in early 1988 of a marked increase of HIV-infected IV drug users in Bangkok. The infection rate in this group went from zero in 1986 to 1 percent in 1987 and 16 percent in early 1988. It is estimated that there are 60,000 IV drug users in Bangkok, and so there may now be close to 10,000 HIV-infected people in that city. Besides posing a great potential for further spread within the IV drug community, these people also provide a relatively large pool for sexual transmission of HIV within that community and outside it.

In Europe the epidemiology of AIDS shows a sharp contrast from east to west and from north to south. In Western Europe the pattern is strikingly similar to that in the U.S., albeit delayed by a couple of years. Homosexual males and IV drug users account for more than 90 percent of AIDS cases, as they do in the U.S.

Regional differences in the share of AIDS cases accounted for by homosexuals and IV drug users are seen in Western Europe, as they are in the U.S. For example, in California homosexual males account for 90 percent of AIDS cases and drug users less than 10 percent; in New York each group accounts for about 50 percent. In such northern countries of

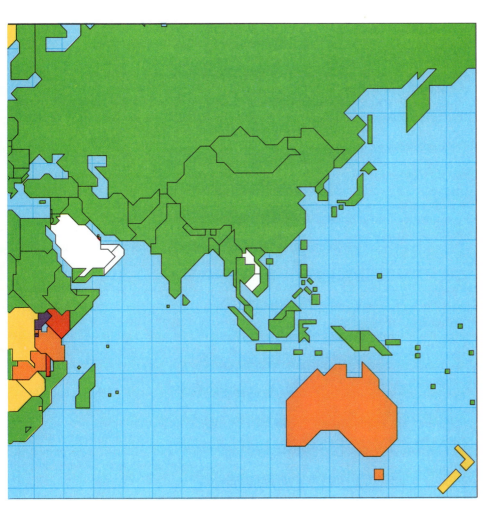

Western Europe as Denmark, Sweden and the U.K., homosexual cases account for from 70 to 90 percent of the total, whereas in two southern countries, Italy and Spain, IV drug users account for more than half of all AIDS cases.

Eastern Europe presents a somewhat different picture. The few AIDS cases that have been reported there collectively represent only about .5 percent of all reported European AIDS cases. Of this small fraction the majority of cases are among homosexual men and IV drug users who have generally acquired their infection from outside Eastern Europe. The delayed appearance of AIDS in Eastern Europe and its low prevalence there compared with Western Europe are likely to be related to different social patterns of homosexuality and to drug use.

The AIDS epidemic in Latin America and the Caribbean, as in the rest of the world, is concentrated primarily in large urban areas. By June of 1988 approximately 8,000 cases had been reported from Latin America and the Caribbean; the number of unreported or unrecognized cases is probably several times this figure. During the first few years of AIDS reporting Latin America followed pattern I: virtually all the reported cases were homosexual men or IV drug users. This was particularly the case in Brazil, where about 3,000 cases have been reported to date, the highest figure from a Latin American country. During the past year or two, however, the trend toward heterosexual acquisition of HIV has been increasing. This is now true in the Caribbean countries of Haiti and the Dominican Republic, where heterosexual cases now outnumber homo-sexual and IV drug cases.

The data that contribute to the preceding epidemiological picture of AIDS enable one to make some broad statements about the present and future. The number of countries reporting to the WHO now stands at 175; 138 have listed at least one AIDS case. As of August 1 these countries had reported 108,176 cases to the WHO Global Program on AIDS. Of these cases about 10,000 were reported in the first half of 1988. Because of inherent delays in reporting as well as the underreporting and under-recognition that persist in many parts of the world, however, a more reasonable estimate of the number of AIDS cases that have already occurred would exceed 250,000.

Estimating the number of HIV-infected people in 1988 is more difficult, because the available se-roprevalence data are limited. As more AIDS testing is carried out and newer studies are made available, estimates will be revised, but the following figures are reasonably conservative.

The U.S. Public Health Service has estimated that between one and 1.5 million people are infected in the U.S. In Europe, epidemiologists responsible for national AIDS surveillance have estimated that by the end of 1987 at least half a million people were infected by HIV. Many serological surveys are still under way in Zaire and Uganda but available data suggest that from two to three million people in Africa may already have been infected by HIV. Adding Canada and Latin America leads one to conclude that a consistent estimate for the minimum number of HIV-infected people worldwide would be five million.

To project the course of AIDS is as difficult as it is important. Many factors complicate accurate prediction of the pandemic's ultimate dimensions: First, it has only been possible to study the scope of the pandemic for about seven years, and there is virtually no other viral infection in human beings whose behavior is similar enough to provide an analogy for predictions. Furthermore, the proportion of HIV-infected individuals who will eventually develop AIDS is still not known. Estimates have ranged from a low of about 10 percent within five years of initial infection to a high of 30 percent or more. Whether the proportion will reach 50, 75 or 100 percent within 10 or 20 years after infection can only be answered with time. The pathogenicity and

distribution of HIV-2 compared with HIV-1 are also not known and need to be determined.

The problem of prediction is complicated by the role of aggravating cofactors of the type already discussed. It has been postulated, for instance, that the presence of other sexually transmitted diseases may facilitate the transmission of HIV. Other cofactors may speed the progression from infection by HIV to the actual development of AIDS, but their roles have not yet been determined. Nor is the degree of infectiousness of HIV-infected people known with any accuracy. Although there is some evidence that infectiousness increases markedly during the later stages of HIV infection, more studies need to be done. Finally, one hopes that current efforts to prevent AIDS will eventually invalidate any long-term prediction based on current data.

In contrast, short-term projections (up to five years) of the number of AIDS cases can be made because they are virtually independent of any future trends in HIV infection. The reason is that the vast majority of the AIDS cases and deaths over the next five years will involve people who are already infected; the cases would develop and the deaths would occur even if all HIV transmission were to cease in 1988. The average period from infection to the development of AIDS is now estimated by most modelers to be between eight and nine years. If five million people are infected worldwide, as estimated above, one can conservatively expect one million new AIDS cases over the next five years. Beyond five years the death toll from those infected as of 1987 could potentially double or triple. We emphasize that this figure does not take into account the number of new infections that will inevitably occur.

The social and economic impact of such an AIDS explosion will be substantial. Mortality rates among the economically and socially most productive age-groups, in particular people from 20 to 49 years old, will rise severalfold in severely affected pattern-I and pattern-II areas as a result of AIDS. This selective impact on young and middle-aged adults, including business and government workers, as well as members of the social, economic and political elites, will have grave economic consequences. The Harvard Institute of International Development estimates that by 1995 the annual loss to Zaire from AIDS' deaths will be $350 million, or 8 percent of the country's 1984 G.N.P.; this was more than Zaire received in that year from all sources of development assistance combined. The same study esti-

COUNTRY	1987 (Cases)	1987 (Rate)	1988 (Cases)
Argentina	51	0.1	43
Australia	342	2.1	143
Austria	85	1.1	37
Bahamas	78	33.9	25
Belgium	85	0.8	25
Brazil	1,361	0.9	206
Burundi	652	13.0	235
Canada	513	1.9	232
Chile	34	0.2	13
Denmark	97	1.8	25
Dominican Republic	256	3.9	152
Ethiopia	19	0.0	18
France	1,852	3.3	555
French Guiana	45	56.2	10
Greece	53	0.5	18
Haiti	332	5.0	231
Honduras	58	1.2	38
Israel	13	0.3	11
Italy	888	1.5	387
Jamaica	37	1.4	13
Japan	34	0.0	7
Mexico	499	0.6	14
Netherlands	215	1.4	75
New Zealand	30	0.9	21
Norway	35	0.8	11
Portugal	44	0.4	35
South Africa	46	0.1	19
Sweden	73	0.8	34
Switzerland	163	2.4	84
United Kingdom	653	1.1	239
United States	21,846	8.9	6,442
West Germany	873	1.4	222
Yugoslavia	18	0.0	12
Zambia	286	4.0	218

Figure 37 ALL COUNTRIES that have reported more than five AIDS cases to the WHO in 1988 are listed here. The left column gives the total number of cases reported by each country for 1987, the middle column gives the 1987 rate (AIDS cases per 100,000 population) and the last column shows the number of cases reported in early 1988. Most 1988 reports were for only the first quarter or third of the year, and so comparison with 1987 should be avoided. Owing to reporting delays of six months or more, cases reported in 1988 actually were diagnosed in 1987. Moreover, some countries with high AIDS rates have not reported any cases in 1988 and so are not shown here.

mates that economic losses in central Africa by 1995 will be $980 million. It is not inconceivable that such social and economic impacts could lead to political destabilization of the countries involved.

The urgency of the situation has resulted in the creation of a global program against AIDS coordinated by the WHO. The program has three objectives: to prevent new HIV infections, to provide support and care to those already infected and to link national and international efforts against AIDS.

The first objective is achievable in principle because it is now known that HIV is almost always transmitted through certain readily identifiable and mostly voluntary behaviors. It is vital to emphasize this point; because they are recognizable, the behaviors that transmit HIV also make it possible to prevent its spread. Consequently information and

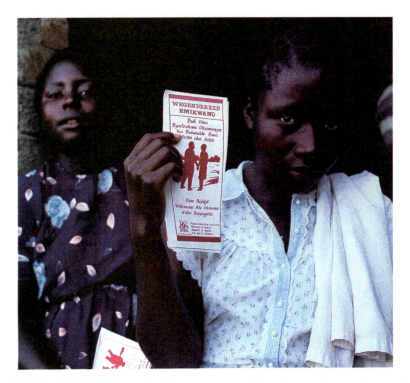

Figure 38 EDUCATIONAL BROCHURES warning Ugandans to "love carefully" and practice "zero grazing" are distributed in 10 languages. The pamphlets held by two girls from the Sese Islands on Lake Victoria follow Ugandan slang in calling AIDS "slim"; this refers to the final stages of the disease, when patients suffer radical weight loss. Since an effective AIDS vaccine is unlikely in the near future, educational measures, now being adopted by dozens of countries, are the only practical way to slow the epidemic.

education programs are needed in all countries. For these education programs to be effective, however, they must be supplemented by health and social services. Advocating the use of condoms is pointless if condoms are not available, costly and of poor quality. Advocating a change of behavior among drug users is fruitless if treatment centers are not available.

Prevention of new HIV infections through blood transfusion is also feasible. Screening of donated blood for HIV antibodies is now routine in the U.S. and in many parts of the industrialized world. In most areas of Africa and Latin America, unfortunately, the cost of screening and the general infrastructure requirements for blood-banking have limited the implementation of such safety measures. Particularly in Africa, voluntary abstention of infected individuals from donating blood or the screening of donors is not likely to protect the blood supply and could drastically reduce the available donor pool. A simple and inexpensive screening assay for HIV infection appropriate for use in the developing world is urgently needed.

The prevention of perinatal transmission depends primarily on protecting women of childbearing age from HIV infection. In women already infected with the virus it may be possible to prevent pregnancy. Dealing with issues of childbearing, contraception and abortion calls for varied approaches adapted to the cultural background of the population.

The second objective of the WHO's global AIDS strategy is to reduce the personal and public impact of HIV infection. This means giving AIDS patients humane care of a quality at least equal to that provided in each society for other diseases. Counseling, social support and services must be available to all infected individuals. HIV-infected persons must not be discriminated against; the rights and dignity of these people must be protected to ensure that AIDS programs can be effective and that the AIDS problem is not simply driven underground.

The third objective, to unify national and international efforts against AIDS, has speedily become a reality. More than 150 countries have now established national AIDS committees. As of June 10, 1988, 151 countries had requested support from the WHO's Global Program on AIDS. Technical evaluation and assessment visits have already taken place in 137 of these countries. Short-term national AIDS plans to cover an initial six-to-18-month period have been established in 106 countries; urgent technical and financial support has been delivered to help start this work without delay. More than 40 countries have been given support to develop medium-term (three-to-five-year) comprehensive na-

tional AIDS plans. Through more than 40 scientific meetings, the WHO has established the basis for national policy formulation; scientific consensus is leading to plans to coordinate international trials of therapeutic agents and AIDS vaccines as these become available for field testing.

There is no precedent in the history of public-health efforts for the speed, intensity or scope of this global mobilization against AIDS. This in itself is cause for optimism. Yet the control and ultimate prevention of AIDS will require sustained, long-term, national and international commitment. There will be no easy answer.

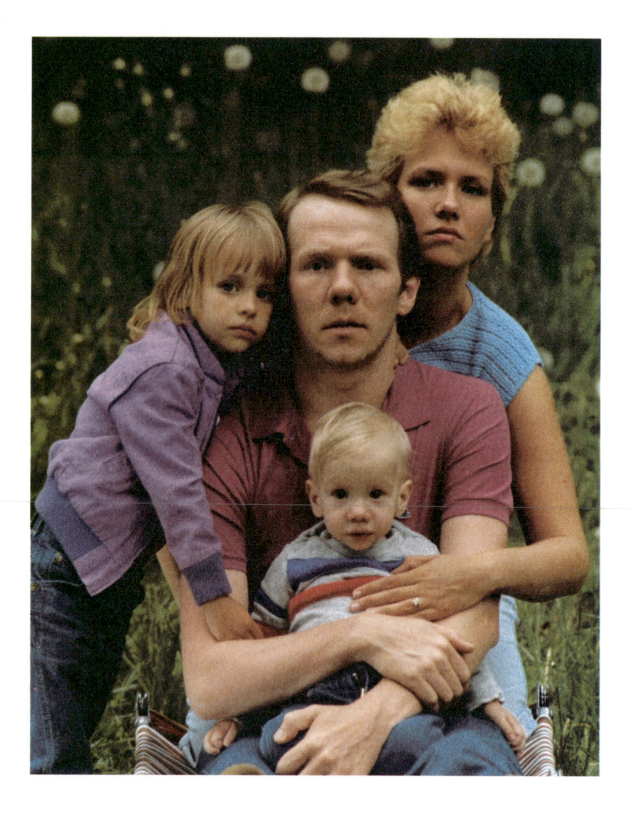

HIV Infection:
The Clinical Picture

The human immunodeficiency virus causes a spectrum of disease that culminates in AIDS. Early detection of HIV infection, often years before symptoms emerge, is the key to prolonging health and life.

. . .

Robert R. Redfield and Donald S. Burke

As physicians we are often asked to describe the typical course of AIDS: the severe immune deficiency that enables normally benign organisms to flourish destructively in patients. Our answer is that people are asking the wrong question. Now that AIDS is known to be caused by a virus—the human immunodeficiency virus, or HIV—the focus should be on the full course of the viral infection, not solely on AIDS. HIV causes a predictable, progressive derangement of immune function, and AIDS is just one, late manifestation of that process.

Figure 39 BURK FAMILY, shown in 1985, looked like a typical U.S. family. Yet the father, Patrick, a hemophiliac, had contracted HIV from a transfusion and, before he was aware of the infection, had passed the virus to his wife, Lauren, who then transmitted it to their son, Dwight, while she was pregnant or breast-feeding. When the photograph was made, Patrick and Dwight already had AIDS; they have since died. The daughter, Nicole, is not infected. There usually are no symptoms of early infection; many people transmit HIV to others before they know they are ill. The authors recommend that anyone who thinks he or she has been exposed to HIV seek an early diagnosis.

An emphasis on HIV is important because it facilitates both treatment and prevention. Prompt diagnosis of HIV infection enables the patient to receive optimal medical care from the earliest moments of the disease. Such care can often prevent complications from developing or getting unnecessarily out of hand. For instance, the lethal opportunistic infection *Pneumocystis carinii* pneumonia (PCP), which has been a hallmark of AIDS, can now actually be prevented with medication given early in the course of HIV disease. (Opportunistic infections are ones that occur because the immune system has broken down.) In addition, the medicine Retrovir (also known as AZT), which has been shown to prolong life in patients with late-stage disease, holds promise as a therapy for patients in earlier stages of infection. Early diagnosis also eliminates the unwitting transmission of HIV and gives people the opportunity to consider changing their behavior before they pass the virus to others.

Although the continuing emphasis on AIDS alone is seriously misguided, it is somewhat understandable. When AIDS was first identified in 1981, it was a mysterious syndrome: a cluster of rare diseases that had suddenly become alarmingly common in homosexual men. In order to identify similar cases of AIDS, and thereby help to uncover the cause and means of transmission, the U.S. Centers for Disease Control (CDC) adopted a strict epidemiological-surveillance definition. People were said to have AIDS if they contracted Kaposi's sarcoma (a rare cancer) or if they developed any of a few rare opportunistic infections, most notably PCP.

The extremely restricted definition worked brilliantly: by 1984 HIV had been identified as the cause of AIDS. Moreover, workers had gained great insight into the methods of transmission, which are now known to be primarily intimate sexual contact, direct contamination of the blood (as when virus-contaminated drug paraphernalia is shared) or the passage of virus from a mother to a fetus or to a suckling baby. Unfortunately the early CDC definition also focused attention so narrowly on AIDS that many doctors and lay people failed to broaden their view once HIV was identified.

Because we and our colleagues at the Walter Reed Army Medical Center believe HIV-infected patients must be treated on the basis of the fullest possible understanding of their disease, in 1984 we developed a classification system that provides a framework for managing patients and understanding the progression of the disease. The system groups patients according to their stage of infection, judged by several indicators of the immune impairment that underlies HIV disease.

As the disease progresses, the patient moves through six stages, the last of which is AIDS. In our system the presence of opportunistic infections is a criterion for the diagnosis of AIDS, but the presence of Kaposi's sarcoma is omitted because the cancer is not caused by immune suppression and can appear early in the course of HIV infection. (Inclusion of Kaposi's sarcoma in the CDC definition hindered the understanding of the natural progression of HIV infection and confounded studies of longevity because patients with Kaposi's sarcoma alone usually lived longer than people who had severe immune impairment.)

The immune dysfunction on which the Walter Reed scheme is based has long been known to result mainly from depletion of a specific set of white blood cells called T4 lymphocytes. The various parts of the immune system are highly interdependent, but if any one part can be called its quarterback, it is the T4 cell, also known as the helper T

cell. Among other functions, it recognizes foreign antigens, or markers, on infected cells and helps to activate another set of white cells called B lymphocytes. The B cells then multiply and produce specific antibodies that bind to infected cells and to free organisms bearing the identified antigen, inactivating those cells and organisms or leading to their destruction. The T4 cell also orchestrates cell-mediated immunity: the killing of infected cells by cytotoxic cells such as T8 lymphocytes and white cells known as natural killer cells.

T4 cells influence the activity of another group of cells as well—the mobile scavengers known as monocytes and macrophages, which engulf infected cells and foreign particles. Activated monocytes and macrophages secrete a variety of cytokines: small but highly potent proteins that modulate the activity of many cell types, including T and B cells. T4 cells also secrete cytokines of their own, notably ones that stimulate the proliferation of T and B cells.

The loss of T4 cells seriously impairs the body's ability to fight most invaders, but it has a particularly severe impact on the defenses against viruses, fungi, parasites and certain bacteria, including mycobacteria (the group that includes the bacterium that causes tuberculosis). Eradication of these organisms requires a strong, highly orchestrated cell-mediated immune response. Other organisms, including many types of bacteria, tend to be destroyed by the "humoral," or antibody-dependent, arm of the immune system. In a humoral response newly made antibodies or antibodies that were stored after an earlier infection attack the invader without T-cell participation. Hence bacterial infections present a smaller threat to people with a limited number of T4 cells.

How exactly does HIV infect and kill T4 cells? Infection begins as a protein, gp120, on the viral envelope binds tightly to a protein known as the CD4 receptor on the cell surface. The virus then merges with the T4 cell and transcribes its RNA genome into double-strand DNA. The viral DNA becomes incorporated into the genetic material in the cell's nucleus and directs the production of new viral RNA and viral proteins, which combine to form new virus particles. These particles bud from the cell membrane and infect other cells.

Early investigations of T4-cell killing demonstrated that under certain circumstances HIV could multiply prodigiously in the helper T cells and kill them, suggesting that viral replication was the main cause of cell destruction. In particular, it was discovered that HIV replication and cell death increase when infected helper *T* cells become activated, as they do when they take part in an immune response to HIV or to other viruses in other cells. Thus the very process that should defeat HIV—an immune response—has the diabolical effect of increasing the proliferation of the virus.

Yet further investigation revealed an apparent paradox: HIV replication could be demonstrated in only a small fraction of *T*4 cells collected from HIV-infected patients. The cells killed by replication alone might hamper the immune system somewhat but would not cause the severe immune deficiency seen in AIDS. The paradox could be resolved only if the cells were also killed by other means. To date several other mechanisms of killing have been documented in the laboratory. Whether they also occur in the body is not yet known. (See Figure 40.)

One mechanism is the formation of syncytia: massive bodies consisting of many merged cells. Syncytia develop after a single cell becomes infected with HIV and produces viral proteins, including gp120, which is displayed on the surface of the infected cell. Because gp120 and the *T*4 cell's CD4 receptor have a high affinity for each other, uninfected *T*4 cells can bind to the infected cell and merge with it. The resulting syncytium cannot function and dies. The original infected cell is killed, but so are dozens or hundreds of uninfected *T*4 cells.

Infected *T*4 cells can also be killed by the standard antiviral activities of cytotoxic antibodies and cells. Even HIV-infected cells that do not produce new virus are vulnerable to immune destruction if they display viral proteins. Similarly, in a process that is unique to HIV, free viral gp120 may circulate in the blood and the lymph and bind to the CD4 receptor of uninfected helper *T* cells, making them susceptible to attack by the immune system.

A final process, which is more speculative, has to do with HIV's effects on cytokine production in various cell types. The virus infects and replicates not only in *T*4 cells but also in monocytes, macrophages and similar cells called tissue-dendritic cells found in the skin, mucous membranes, lymph nodes, liver, spleen and brain. Such cells are not killed by the virus, but their functioning may nonetheless be deranged in some ways. In particular, HIV infection may somehow alter the amount or structure of the cytokines normally produced by activated macrophages or activated lymphocytes in a way that is toxic to helper *T* cells.

Regardless of how helper *T* cells are killed by HIV, their progressive decline leads to a more general decline in immune functioning and hence is the primary factor determining the clinical course of the patient. In recognition of those cells' importance, the Walter Reed classification system relies on the *T*4-cell count and function as an indicator of a patient's stage of disease. Other indicators include the onset of chronic lymphadenopathy, or swollen lymph nodes, the response to a set of skin tests that reflect the overall functioning of cell-mediated immunity and the presence of infections that have been unequivocally associated with a specific degree of immune suppression. Lymphadenopathy and abnormal test results must persist for at least three months before they are taken to be evidence of the stage of infection.

The specific stages chart the course of the immune system's decline. When HIV infection is first detectable by standard tests, the *T*4-cell concentration is often close to the normal level of about 800 cells per cubic millimeter of blood, and the patient feels well. Usually within six months to a year, chronic lymphadenopathy develops. Within a few years laboratory and other tests reveal more severe, subclinical (silent) immune defects: first the slowly declining *T*4-cell count falls below 400 and then patients exhibit abnormalities on the skin tests. Later, as the *T*4-cell number drops further, overt disease sets in, first as chronic infections of the skin and mucous membranes and then as disseminated, systemic infections.

Throughout the course of HIV infection people may also develop cancers and disorders of the central nervous system. These are noted along with the Walter Reed stage of disease but are not included in the criteria for each stage because in most instances their causes and their relation to the immune deficiency are not known. The same is true for the various "constitutional" symptoms that some physicians have dubbed the AIDS-related complex, or ARC: unexplained fevers, persistent night sweats, chronic diarrhea and wasting. We hope the data we are collecting about all these disorders and their relation to the stage of disease will lead to new insights into their causes and to new treatments.

The Walter Reed classification system (see Figure 41) begins with stage zero: exposure to the virus through any of the known transmission routes. Noting exposure facilitates early diagnosis: people who are known to have been exposed to HIV can be

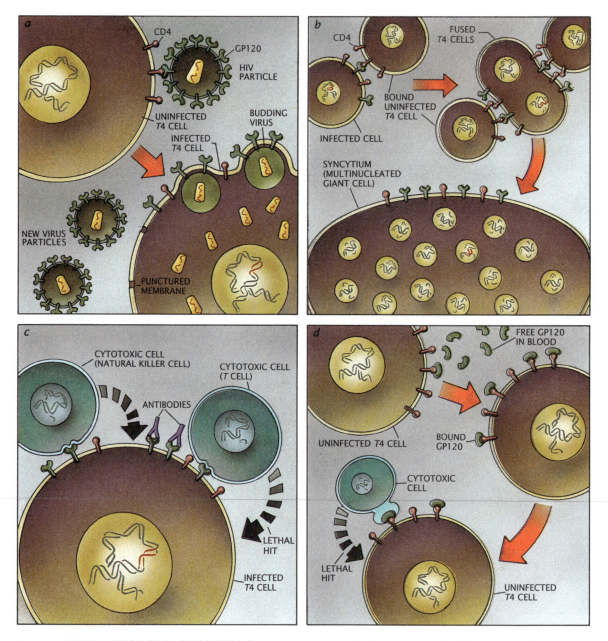

Figure 40 DESTRUCTION OF *T*4 CELLS. HIV is known to kill cells by replicating, budding from them and damaging the cell membrane (*a*). HIV might also kill *T*4 cells indirectly, by means of a viral protein, gp120, that is displayed on an infected cell's surface. A molecule on *T*4 cells—the CD4 receptor—has a strong affinity for gp120, and healthy *T*4 cells can bind to the gp120 and merge with the infected cell (*b*). The end result, called a syncytium, cannot survive, and all the once healthy cells it contains are destroyed along with the infected cell. HIV can also elicit normal cellular immune defenses against infected cells (*c*). With or without the help of antibodies, cytotoxic defensive cells can destroy an infected cell that displays viral proteins on its surface. Finally, free gp120 may circulate in the blood of people with HIV (*d*). The free protein may bind to the CD4 receptor of uninfected cells, making them appear to be infected and evoking an immune response.

STAGE	HIV ANTIBODY AND/OR VIRUS	CHRONIC LYMPHAD- ENOPATHY	T-HELPER CELLS/MM^3	DELAYED HYPER- SENSITIVITY	THRUSH	OPPORTUNISTIC INFECTIONS
WR0	−	−	> 400	NORMAL	−	−
WR1	+	−	> 400	NORMAL	−	−
WR2	+	+	> 400	NORMAL	−	−
WR3	+	+/−	< 400	NORMAL	−	−
WR4	+	+/−	< 400	P	−	−
WR5	+	+/−	< 400	C AND/OR THRUSH		−
WR6	+	+/−	< 400	P/C	+/−	+

Figure 41 WALTER REED CLASSIFICATION SYSTEM charts the course of patients from exposure to HIV (WR0) and the onset of infection (WR1) through stages of progressive immune dysfunction. The essential criteria by which patients are assigned to each stage are shown in red and always include laboratory evidence of HIV infection. Under "Delayed Hypersensitivity" P indicates a partial defect and C refers to complete failure to respond to the skin tests. Patients enter stage 6 and are said to have AIDS when opportunistic infections (ones that occur because the immune system has broken down), such as cryptococcal meningitis, develop elsewhere in the body.

evaluated for evidence of infection, such as the presence of antibodies to HIV in the blood. Even before infection is detected they can be told that they may be infected with HIV and so should take steps to avoid spreading the possible infection to others; HIV usually causes no symptoms at first and can take root from six weeks to a year before it is detected by the standard (antibody) HIV test. Stage zero has also been included to emphasize the fact that, in 1988, exposure to HIV, rather than membership in some "risk" group, is the single most important factor leading to HIV infection.

Once the presence of HIV has been documented by any reliable test, patients are said to be in Walter Reed stage 1, provided they do not meet the criteria for a higher stage. In addition to identifying antibodies to HIV in blood samples, some laboratories are now able to detect infection by culturing whole virus or identifying viral nucleic acid or protein in blood or tissue samples.

Although most people have no symptoms when HIV infection is first diagnosed, some patients develop a disorder resembling mononucleosis. Its symptoms include fatigue, fever and swollen glands, which may or may not be accompanied by a rash. In addition self-limited disorders of the central nervous system have been noted. These range from headaches to encephalitis (inflammation of brain tissue). The cause of these symptoms is not entirely clear. In any event, they disappear, usually within a few weeks. Unfortunately HIV does not do the same; it continues to replicate and slowly but persistently destroys T4 cells.

For the majority of patients the first sign that something is amiss in the immune system is the development of chronically swollen lymph nodes. With the appearance of this chronic lymphadenopathy a patient moves into stage 2. The cause of the lymphadenopathy is relatively straightforward. Although HIV infection suppresses many immune functions, it also is marked by one kind of hyperactivity. The ongoing presence of HIV overstimulates B cells, which are abundant in the lymph nodes, and keeps them in a state of chronic activation. The flood of antibodies produced as a result of such activation includes some antibodies that combat current infections or recurrences of past infections. In general, however, the hyperactivity is not beneficial. The activation of large numbers of B cells diminishes the number of resting cells that can differentiate to produce antibodies in response to new pathogens or to inoculation with vaccines.

Stage 2 typically lasts for from three to five years, and patients still feel well even when it ends. The beginning of stage 3 is defined by a persistent drop in the T4-cell count to less than 400, which is a harbinger of a decline in immune functioning. Patients remain in this stage, however, until direct evidence of an impairment in cell-mediated immunity is discovered—usually about 18 months later—at which point they enter stage 4. That evidence is the failure to respond to three out of four skin tests that measure what is called delayed hypersensitivity: the individual's ability to mount a cellular immune response against specific proteins injected under the skin.

Although the T4-cell count in stage 4 can dip quite low (for example, to 50), the Walter Reed system requires only that it be persistently less than 400 in this stage and also in stages 5 and 6. This criterion is not narrower, because patients can vary quite a bit in their immune function at any specific low T4-cell count.

Progression to stage 5 is usually determined on the basis of the development of anergy (a total absence of delayed hypersensitivity). Some time later the first overt symptom of a breakdown in cell-mediated immunity arises: the development of thrush, a fungal infection of the mucous membranes of the tongue or the oral cavity. Thrush, which can occasionally develop before anergy, is identified by the presence of white spots and ulcers covering the infected area. By the time most people reach stage 5, their T4-cell count has generally fallen to less than 200.

In addition to thrush, stage-5 patients often develop unusually severe or persistent viral or fungal infections of the skin and mucous membranes. One example is chronic infection with the Herpes simplex virus, which often produces painful and persistent sores in the skin surrounding the anus, the genital area or the mouth. In addition, *Candida albicans*, the fungus that causes thrush, may spread throughout the vagina, resulting in chronic infection there.

Recently many stage-5 patients have developed oral hairy leukoplakia: a mucous-membrane infection marked by fuzzy white patches, usually on the tongue, that cannot be rubbed off. The cause is not clear. Although these infections now appear to be the commonest ones in stage 5, it is becoming apparent that any viral or fungal pathogen in the skin or mucous membranes can cause equally severe infection at this stage of the immune deficiency.

Many people develop chronic or disseminated opportunistic infections at sites beyond the skin and mucous membranes within a year or two after entering stage 5. The emergence of these infections reflects an extremely severe decline in immune function and constitutes progression to stage 6, or what is also called opportunistic-infection-defined AIDS. (Again, Kaposi's sarcoma is not sufficient evidence of stage-6 disease.) Most patients enter stage 6 with a T4-cell count of 100 or less and most, unfortunately, die within two years.

We cannot discuss all of the many opportunistic infections that can develop during stage 6, but we shall mention a few that are particularly common or virulent in the U.S. The diseases that appear most often in this stage—and in stage 5—are prevalent probably because the agents that cause them are ubiquitous in human beings. Similarly, infections that appear in some geographic areas but not in others are probably caused by organisms that are prevalent in distinct locales. We should also point out that any pathogen that can be eradicated only with the help of vigorous cell-mediated immunity can cause serious disease. Hence, in addition to the exotic infections that receive most of the publicity, a host of more familiar diseases, such as tuberculosis, can also develop and be quite severe.

In addition to PCP, other disorders associated with AIDS include the parasitic infections toxoplasmosis (which often infects the brain and can lead to seizures and coma) and chronic cryptosporidiosis (which typically attacks the intestinal tract, causing chronic diarrhea). Stage-6 opportunistic diseases also include the fungal infections cryptococcosis (which frequently causes meningitis but may also damage the liver, bone, skin and other tissues) and histoplasmosis (which can cause self-limited pneumonia in individuals with an intact immune system but causes a disseminated infection of the liver, bone marrow and other tissues in HIV-infected patients and is a frequent cause of chronic fevers).

A common viral infection is cytomegalovirus, a cause of pneumonia, encephalitis, blindness and inflammation of the gastrointestinal tract. As is the case with histoplasmosis and tuberculosis, the cytomegalovirus infection seen in HIV patients is usually a reactivation of a childhood infection that was well controlled until HIV seriously hobbled the patient's immune system. Such bacteria as *Legionella*

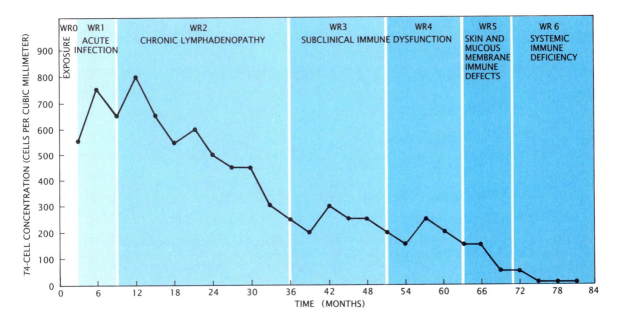

Figure 42 DECLINE in *T*4-cell count (rounded to the nearest 50) was tracked in the blood of a young man whose disease followed a typical course. About three months after sexual exposure to HIV the patient tested positive for the virus; his *T*4-cell count dropped and then rebounded. He developed chronic lymphadenopathy at nine months and, at 51 months, after a long, slow decline in his *T*4-cell count, exhibited chronic, subtle abnormalities of delayed hypersensitivity. He displayed persistent anergy at 63 months but had no overt symptoms of infection until about 68 months, when he developed thrush and oral hairy leukoplakia. Less than a year later he was besieged by opportunistic infections, including cytomegalovirus infection, which made him blind. He died at 83 months.

and *Salmonella* can also be a severe problem for someone in stage 6.

Standard or experimental therapies exist for all these disorders. Among the most exciting developments in recent years is the discovery of several medications that control or even prevent PCP. Pentamidine, Septra/Bactrium and dapsone are all effective in clearing up the infection; the first two — and a drug called Fansidar — serve as preventives as well.

Also exciting are new treatments for cytomegalovirus. Just two years ago investigators had little hope of discovering an effective therapy for the virus. Today there are two treatments, including a medicine (ganciclovir) that can halt the progression of cytomegalovirus-induced blindness. Research workers are making progress against other HIV-related diseases as well. A drug called acyclovir is under study for the prevention of Herpes simplex infection, and new treatments have been developed for cryptococcal meningitis, disseminated histoplasmosis and mycobacterial diseases.

Just as investigators continue to seek better treatments for the opportunistic infections associated with HIV, so too the search continues for the causes of the neurological disorders and cancers that have been associated with HIV infection. Thus far the causes — and their relation to immune deficiency — are a matter of conjecture. One would expect that conditions arising late in the course of infection could be a consequence of immune deficiency, whereas conditions arising earlier would probably have other causes.

Early neurological findings can include subtle alterations in cognitive function, such as in memory and judgment. The brain damage could stem from diseases that are transmitted in the same way as HIV, such as syphilis, and that often coexist with it. On the other hand, HIV may cause trouble on its own, for example by replicating in brain cells or inducing the secretion of neurotoxic cytokines.

In the terminal stages of HIV infection many patients suffer from the AIDS dementia complex: a syndrome characterized by a gradual loss of precision

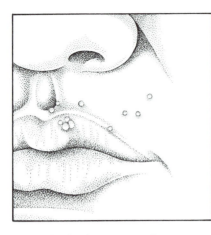

Figure 43 VIRAL INFECTION known as molluscum contagiosum normally produces a few small lesions (*left*) that disappear on their own within several months. In a patient with advanced HIV infection the lesions persisted, grew and multiplied so profusely (*right*) that they disfigured the face, demonstrating that when the immune system is compromised, even common, ordinarily minor infections can be overwhelming.

in both thought and motion. In the end, some people are unable to walk or communicate effectively. The cause remains a mystery.

The cancers associated with HIV are also perplexing. In addition to Kaposi's sarcoma, which produces tumors in the skin and in the linings of internal organs, they include various lymphomas (cancers of lymphoid tissue) and cancers of the rectum and tongue. Some workers have postulated that Kaposi's sarcoma is caused in part by HIV-induced changes in the amounts or types of cytokines produced by defensive cells or by other cell types. These changes could occur quite early and could explain why Kaposi's sarcoma often appears relatively early in the course of HIV infection.

Certain lymphomas can also develop quite early, lending credence to the notion that B-cell hyperactivity plays a role in their development. Lymphomas that arise later might result from cancer-causing viruses that take hold in the course of immune deficiency. If the immune system provides constant surveillance against cancer, as dogma says it does, the lymphomas and other cancers that appear late in HIV disease could also stem from the failure of the compromised immune system to recognize and destroy cancer cells.

We expect that looking at cancers and neurological disorders within the framework of the Walter Reed classification system will help to distinguish those that stem from immune dysfunction from those that arise by other means. On another front, the system has made it possible to show that most people infected with HIV follow about the same basic course and do indeed move from stage to stage. The notion that genetic variation in the virus or distinctive features of the patient are the crucial factors influencing the disease course has now fallen by the wayside.

Early studies of disease progression by other investigators were relatively optimistic, suggesting that only about 30 to 40 percent of patients infected with HIV progressed to AIDS. Without a staging system, however, such studies could not say whether the remaining subjects progressed to some intermediate stage of disease.

In contrast, early diagnosis of HIV infection and the use of the Walter Reed system has been standard practice in the U.S. military services for several years (thanks to enlightened military leadership and extraordinary commitment and cooperation among an array of health professionals). The primary aim has been to facilitate optimal medical care and prevention, but proper diagnosis combined with accurate staging has also provided information about the natural history of HIV infection in young adults. In addition to diagnosing more than 5,000 individuals with HIV, military physicians have tracked the course of some 900 of those patients for more than a year, a subset of some 250 patients for more than 18 months and a smaller subset of about 60 patients for more than three years (see Figure 44).

Looking at progression by one or more stages and not just at the development of AIDS, we have found that the longer we follow our patients, the greater the percentage is of people who progress to a higher stage. Whereas 54 percent of the patients in the group followed for one year remained in their initial stage at the end of the study period, only about 8 percent of the smaller, three-year group stayed in the same stage. In other words, more than 90 percent of the patients progressed within three years.

When we looked at the progression to stage 6 (opportunistic-infection-defined AIDS), we found that after three years 10 percent of the patients initially in Walter Reed stage 2, 29 percent of those in stage 3, 71 percent of those in stage 4 and 100 percent of those in stage 5 had moved into stage 6 or had died. These findings underscore the grim reality that, in the absence of a scientific solution to HIV, most (and perhaps all) people who are infected with HIV will eventually develop end-stage disease and will die prematurely.

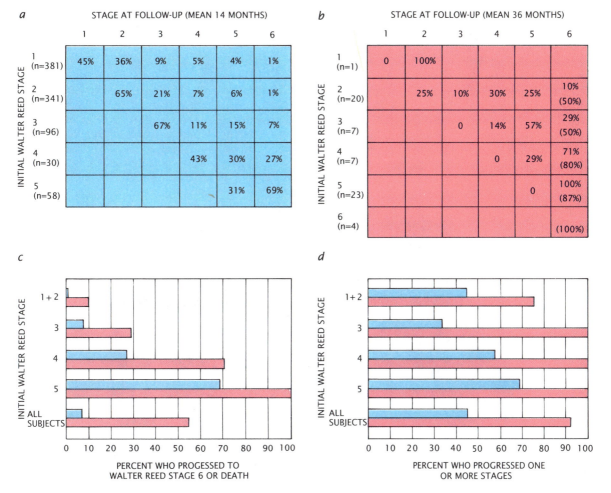

Figure 44 DISEASE PROGRESSION was examined in 906 patients followed for a mean of 14 months (*a*) and in a subset of 62 patients followed for a mean of 36 months (*b*). (Numbers in parentheses reflect the percentage of stage-6 patients who died.) Comparison of the percentage of patients who moved from their initial Walter Reed stage to stage 6 (*c*) or who progressed by one or more stages (*d*)

revealed that the longer people with HIV are followed, the more likely it is they will have moved to a severer stage of disease. For example, the shorter study (*pink*) found that about half of the subjects advanced one or more stages by the end of the follow-up period, but the longer study (*blue*) found that more than 90 percent of subjects had advanced.

One question relating to disease progression remains: Why is it that the disease progresses slowly? One theory holds that the answer lies with the virus alone. For instance, HIV might be a slow-replicating organism that initially poses little danger to cells but later changes into a more active and highly cytotoxic agent. Another theory postulates that HIV is active in the body throughout the infection but its cytotoxic effects are held in check for a time by the immune system. Although viral factors likely play some role, the activity of the immune system is probably of paramount importance.

One reason we think so is that a range of defensive activities have been shown to occur after infection with HIV, demonstrating that the body initially mounts a vigorous immune response. These activities include the production of different types of antibodies against the virus — some that neutralize it, others that prevent it from binding to cells and still others that stimulate cytotoxic cells to attack infected cells. The response also includes direct activation of the cellular arm of the immune system.

Such findings suggest that the immune system limits viral replication for quite some time but that the potent virus slowly gains ground. Eventually a threshold is reached (probably between stages 3 and 5): the decline in $T4$ cells is so significant that the immune system can no longer function efficiently enough to hold HIV in check. Viral proliferation increases, as does the virus's toxicity, and the balance of power shifts in favor of the virus. With time the decline in $T4$ cells is so severe that the immune system becomes essentially nonfunctional. Then the virus proliferates wildly, destroying the $T4$ cells that remain in the body.

This model postulates a gradual rise in the amount of virus in the blood with time, rather than a steady, low level followed by a sudden rise. Indeed, with each successive stage of disease the amount of viral protein that can be detected increases, as does the ability to isolate virus from the blood.

The implications of these observations go far beyond proving the validity of a theoretical model. More virus in the body means greater infectivity. Indeed, we in the military, and workers elsewhere, have demonstrated that as the $T4$-cell depletion progresses, an infected person's likelihood of trans-

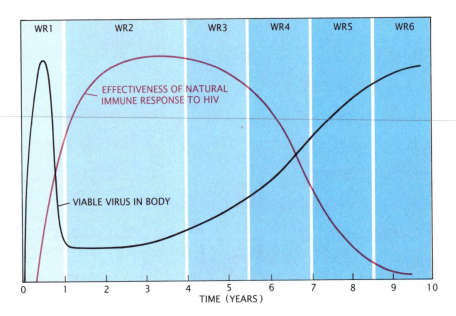

Figure 45 BALANCE OF POWER between HIV (*black curve*) and the immune system (*red curve*) shifts during the course of the infection, according to a model proposed by the authors. The amount of HIV in the body soars in the first days of infection, but once the immune system "kicks in," it initially operates normally and reduces the amount of virus. The immune system remains in good control of the virus for several years, but HIV gains ground slowly. At some point the $T4$ cells that orchestrate the immune response become so depleted that the balance of power switches. HIV then replicates wildly, killing the remaining $T4$ cells and hence any vestiges of immune defense.

mitting the disease to a spouse increases. Hence the longer people are infected with HIV and the more immune-deficient they become, the more readily they seem to pass HIV to others. People are also likely to be highly infectious at the earliest moments of infection, before the immune system "kicks in" effectively, and particularly before antibodies are detected.

These findings highlight, once again, the importance of medical follow-up and early diagnosis of HIV infection for anyone who has been exposed to the virus, including people who have been in a long-term sexual relationship. Only with such follow-up can physicians undertake the public-health measures, and patients undertake the personal measures, needed to prevent the spread of the disease.

Our report here is less optimistic than many people would wish. Yet we are not discouraged, nor should they be. HIV infection may seem in 1988 to be insurmountable, but it is important to put the current situation in perspective. When the father of one of us (Redfield) was a physician, there was no effective therapy for bacterial diseases. Young children were almost certain to die when they developed rather common bacterial infections such as periorbital cellulitis, which affects the skin and soft tissue around the eyes. He had to have the courage to tell the parents of those children that, although he would do his best, in the end their seemingly healthy child would almost certainly die. This was so in the late 1930's; it was so in the early 1940's. Yet by the late 1940's his practice required a little less courage. With the advent of penicillin, he had a new and important tool for treating bacterial infections. Today most young children with periorbital cellulitis survive.

We do not pretend that HIV will be defeated easily, but doctors and patients should keep in sight the day when medical science will reduce HIV infection to a curable disease. We have no doubt that day will come. In the study of new diseases there must first be a time when physicians can only describe symptoms and treat patients with whatever seems to work best. Then comes an understanding of causation and of the disease's natural course, which enables physicians to provide patients with an early diagnosis and accurate clinical assessment. Next comes the development of effective treatments based on the new knowledge, and then refinement of treatments until a cure is found.

Investigators are completing the descriptive phase and are fully immersed in understanding the hows and whys of the virus. If we persist and are methodical, we shall unquestionably succeed in curing HIV infection.

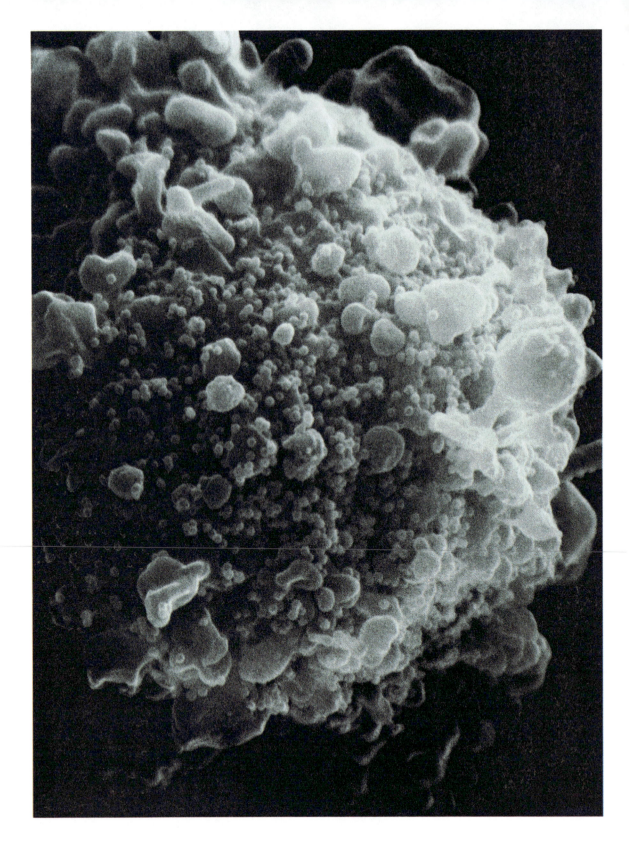

HIV Infection:
The Cellular Picture

*A key finding of AIDS research is that infection begins when
HIV binds to a molecule called CD4 on the target cell. Knowledge of
that interaction may help in developing therapies or vaccines.*

• • •

Jonathan N. Weber and Robin A. Weiss

Like all viruses, the human immunodeficiency virus (HIV) is an intracellular parasite: the virus particle itself is inert and cannot propagate or do any damage until it enters a host cell. How does the virus actually enter the cell? The answer will help investigators to understand the clinical course of AIDS, the disease caused by the virus. More than that, an understanding of how HIV enters cells may eventually make it possible to develop vaccines or protective medications that can block the action of HIV at the earliest possible stage: before it infects its first host cells.

The first step in any viral infection is the binding of the virus particle to a component of the host cell's membrane. In the case of HIV, workers have found that the virus binds to the molecule known as the CD4 antigen. (An antigen is a molecule that can be recognized by an antibody.) Hence the distribution of CD4 in the body reflects the tropism of HIV: the kinds of cells and tissues the virus infects and destroys. The CD4 antigen is found primarily on cells of the immune system called helper T cells (although other kinds of cells also carry it); HIV infection is characterized by the loss of these cells, which causes a deterioration of the immune system.

For some time it has been known that the binding takes place when CD4 interacts with an "envelope" protein of the virus called gp120 (because it is a glycoprotein—a protein containing sugar complexes—with a molecular weight of 120 kilodaltons) that is distributed on the outside of the viral membrane. Investigators are now identifying the specific portions of the CD4 and gp120 molecules that take part in the binding interaction. Such knowledge makes it possible to envisage a two-pronged attack on HIV: denying access to the cellular CD4 receptor, both by covering up the viral gp120 protein and by blocking the receptor.

Figure 46 INFECTED *T* CELL (a cell of the immune system) produces particles (*small spheres*) of the human immunodeficiency virus (HIV) in this image. The scanning electron micrograph shows part of the infected cell's convoluted surface, magnified about 20,000 diameters. (Micrograph by David Hockley of the National Institute for Biological Standards and Control in England.)

The chain of experiments that eventually identified CD4 as the molecule to which HIV binds began in June, 1984, when samples of the virus became generally available for research. In one of the earliest experiments, Mika Popovic of the National Institutes of Health studied the growth of HIV in fresh peripheral-blood lymphocytes (white blood cells freshly separated from the bloodstream) and in lines of tumor cells that are able to grow perpetually in culture. He found that HIV grew best in a line of leukemic T cells. (The T cells, a major class of cells in the immune system, include the helper T cells and cells called cytotoxic, or killer, T cells.)

At about the same time, David Klatzmann of the Salpêtrière Hospital in Paris noted that in fresh peripheral-blood lymphocytes infected in culture with HIV there was a decrease in the number of cells bearing the CD4 antigen; the decrease was paralleled by an increase in the HIV replication rate. Klatzmann then divided the T cells from a sample of peripheral-blood lymphocytes into T-helper and T-cytotoxic subsets. He found that only helper T cells—the cells that bear the CD4 antigen—supported the replication of HIV. Klatzmann's findings dovetailed well with an observation made in 1981 in the first published clinical description of AIDS patients. In that report Michael S. Gottlieb of the University of California at Los Angeles School of Medicine had noted that lymphocytes bearing CD4 were reduced in number or absent entirely from the blood of AIDS patients.

Simultaneously in London, Angus G. Dalgleish and Paul R. Clapham in our laboratory at the Institute of Cancer Research tackled the question of the tropism of HIV from another direction. We tested antibodies to various cell-surface antigens to see which of them would block molecules crucial to the binding of the virus. In these experiments we first exposed susceptible T cells to the antibodies and then to virus particles. Next we applied various assays to determine how the antibodies had affected HIV's ability to infect the cells. These experiments revealed that monoclonal antibodies (antibodies that bind only to a single, specific molecular target) to the CD4 antigen, but not those to other cell-surface antigens, could block the infectivity of HIV. Klatzmann, using different assays, got similar results.

Another kind of assay took advantage of a sign of HIV infection we had noted in cell cultures: the formation of "multinucleated syncytia." These are giant cells consisting of several nuclei contained within a single membrane; they form when HIV-infected cells fuse with healthy cells bearing the receptor molecules. We found that antibodies to CD4 could indeed block the formation of syncytia.

Still another assay for receptors, first developed for work on animal retroviruses by Jan Zavada of the Institute of Virology in Bratislava, is known as a pseudotype assay. This method involves exposing cells that have already been infected with HIV to a second, unrelated virus called vesicular stomatitis virus (VSV). VSV is a plaque-forming virus: it causes the formation of visible plaques made up of dead cells. When HIV-infected cells are "superinfected" with VSV, they produce a number of virus particles that have the envelope proteins of HIV but the genetic material and plaque-forming properties of VSV. These "transvestite" particles are called VSV(HIV) pseudotypes. Because the pseudotypes have the same envelope characteristics as HIV, they recognize the same receptors and enter the target cell in the same way; their ability to infect particular cells should therefore parallel that of HIV. After they enter the cell, however, they replicate as VSV and form plaques. Hence the appearance of plaques in various kinds of cells indicates the presence on the surface of those cells of the receptor for HIV.

Dalgleish and his colleagues noted that VSV(HIV) pseudotypes would form plaques only among cells bearing the CD4 antigen. Furthermore, the antibodies to CD4 that blocked the formation of syncytia also prevented the formation of plaques.

Subsequently J. Steven McDougal of the Centers for Disease Control in Atlanta (CDC) devised a physical assay for determining whether HIV particles had attached to cells; he found that HIV would bind only to cells bearing the CD4 antigen and, once again, that binding could be inhibited by anti-CD4 monoclonal antibodies. McDougal also showed that gp120 molecules attached to antibodies could draw CD4 molecules from a preparation of cell-membrane material. All these experiments suggested that the CD4 antigen—the disappearance of which had been part of the clinical definition of AIDS from the disease's earliest days—is itself the receptor for HIV.

The strongest evidence that CD4 is the receptor for HIV came in 1986 from Paul Maddon and Richard Axel of the Columbia University College of Physicians and Surgeons. They transferred the gene that encodes the CD4 molecule into HeLa cells, a line of cervical-cancer cells that do not make CD4 and cannot ordinarily be infected with HIV. Maddon and Axel found that the altered, CD4-bearing HeLa cells could now be infected with HIV; when they were infected, they rapidly fused into giant syncytia. Expression of the CD4 gene was enough to confer susceptibility to HIV.

This experiment led to one unexpected result, which has not yet been explained fully. Maddon, working in collaboration with Clapham and Dalgleish in London and McDougal at the CDC, transfected the human CD4 gene into mouse T cells; the cells then produced human CD4. HIV particles bound to these altered cells, but there was no evidence that the cells actually became infected: no syncytia were formed and no infectious virus was produced. This was surprising, because mouse cells can indeed produce HIV under certain conditions; for example, Jay A. Levy of the University of California at San Francisco School of Medicine and other investigators successfully transfected the entire HIV genome into mouse cells, which then produced infectious virus. Apparently, however, mouse cells cannot be infected by free HIV particles, even in the presence of the HIV receptor. Even VSV(HIV) pseudotypes were unable to infect them, although VSV, once it enters mouse cells, can usu-

ally replicate perfectly well. These results suggest another component of the cell surface is required for the virus to achieve full entry after it has bound to the cell membrane. The nature of this second factor is not known.

The binding of viral gp120 to cellular CD4 is only the first step of viral entry into the cell. The later steps have been less thoroughly elucidated. For example, how does the virus's genetic material enter the cell? The simplest and likeliest possibility is that the viral membrane simply fuses with the cell membrane, injecting the core of the virus (including its genetic material) into the cell. Another possibility is that the cell membrane forms a small pocket that later becomes an enclosed sac called an endocytic vesicle. The vesicle completely surrounds the virus particle and carries it into the cell. Then a reaction within the cell acidifies the membrane of which the vesicle (now called an endosome) is made. When the endosome is acidified, it undergoes a conformational change and fuses with the viral membrane, releasing the viral core into the cell's interior.

Recent evidence casts doubt on the relevance of this mechanism, which is known as receptor-mediated endocytosis. Barry S. Stein of the Stanford University School of Medicine and Myra O.

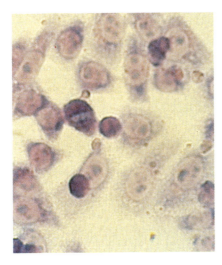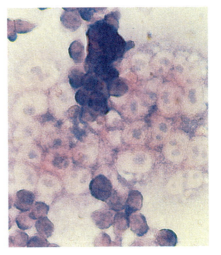

Figure 47 MULTINUCLEATED SYNCYTIA, clusters of many nuclei within a single cell membrane, are a sign of HIV infection in cell cultures. They form when infected cells, which make gp120 and carry it on their surface, fuse with healthy cells bearing the CD4 molecule. The photograph at the left shows HeLa cells, a line of cervical-cancer cells that do not make the CD4 molecule and cannot be infected with HIV. They have been exposed to HIV, but no syncytia have formed. The photograph at the right shows HeLa cells that have been genetically altered so that they make the CD4 molecule. These cells, on being exposed to HIV, have become infected and have formed syncytia.

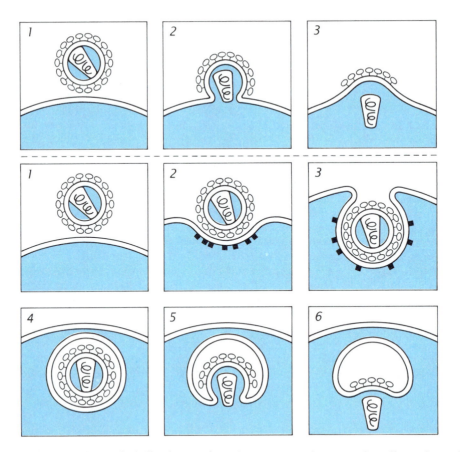

Figure 48 ENTRY of the virus's core, including its genetic material, into the target cell probably takes place by one of two mechanisms. The likeliest (*top*) is direct fusion. In this mechanism the virus particle binds to the cell (*1*) and the viral membrane fuses with the cell membrane (*2*), ejecting the core material into the cell (*3*). The other mechanism (*bottom*), called receptor-mediated endocytosis, also begins when the virus particle binds to the cell membrane (*1*). In the next stage, however, the cell membrane buckles inward to form a pocket (*2*) known as a coated pit. The membrane encloses the virus particle (*3*) and detaches from the cell surface to form a body called an endosome (*4*). Eventually the viral membrane fuses with the membrane of the endosome (*5*), releasing the viral core into the interior of the cell (*6*).

McClure of our laboratory have shown independently that the entry of HIV into the cell is independent of acidity: drugs that block the acidification of endosomes do not prevent HIV infection. In addition, Dan R. Littman of San Francisco and Maddon have shown that mutations in the "tail" of the CD4 antigen (the part within the cell) that prevent the antigen's incorporation into endosomes do not inhibit HIV infection. It is likely, then, that HIV enters the cell by fusing directly with the cell membrane.

The direct-fusion mechanism would also help to explain the cell-to-cell fusion that leads to the formation of syncytia. Syncytia form because HIV-infected cells manufacture gp120 and carry it on their cell membrane. When an infected cell meets a healthy cell that bears the CD4 antigen, the gp120 of the infected cell can bind to the CD4 of the healthy cell. Then the two cells join, probably by direct fusion. The resulting syncytium continues to carry gp120 on its cell membrane, and so it can continue to fuse with healthy cells. One infected cell may eventually bring together as many as 50 cells.

In any case, whether direct fusion or receptor-mediated endocytosis is the correct model, the viral

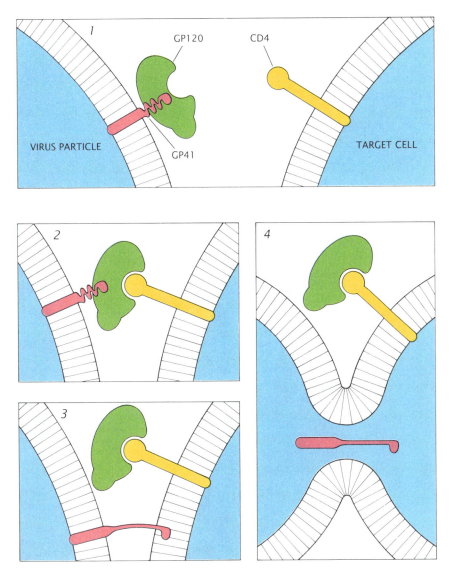

Figure 49 BINDING of a virus particle to a target cell depends on an interaction between a molecule on the surface of the virus and a molecule on the membrane of the target cell. As the virus approaches the cell (*1*), a viral protein designated gp120 binds to a cell-surface molecule known as CD4 (*2*). That interaction uncovers another protein called gp41. One end of the gp41 molecule embeds itself in the cell membrane (*3*), leading to the eventual fusion of the viral membrane and the cell membrane (*4*).

membrane must fuse with a membrane of the cell. How does that happen? According to a plausible model, the binding of gp120 to CD4 causes a change in the shape of the gp120 protein, revealing a part of another envelope protein, known as gp41, that is normally hidden under the gp120 molecule. This region of gp41 is hydrophobic: it will embed itself in a cell membrane rather than remaining exposed to the aqueous solution surrounding the cell. Once it is uncovered, the hydrophobic region of gp41 interacts with the adjacent cell membrane and induces the viral membrane and the cell membrane to fuse together. It is not clear whether some receptor on the cell surface other than the CD4 antigen binds to gp41 or whether gp41 embeds itself directly in the cell membrane.

After HIV enters the cell, its genetic material, which is encoded in RNA, is converted into DNA. The DNA "provirus" is then integrated into the DNA of the target cell. This means that the infection is persistent for the cell's lifetime and that of its progeny if it multiplies. The integrated virus may remain completely "silent," or else it may manifest itself in any one of at least three ways.

First, the viral genome may cause a persistent infection, in which some new virus particles are created but few cells are killed. Second, infection may lead to the creation of syncytia, which die soon after forming. Syncytia are a dominant effect of HIV infection in cell culture. In human beings they are sometimes seen (particularly in the brain) during later stages of infection, but it is not clear whether they play a role in the early pathogenesis of AIDS.

A third possible result of HIV infection is the rapid death of cells without the formation of syncytia. It is not yet known how HIV kills cells. Perhaps some product encoded by the HIV genes is directly toxic. Alternatively, perhaps the gp120 that is made and embedded in cell membranes as a result of infection binds to CD4 that is already there; such binding could damage the cell's membrane systems. The host's immune response also shapes the fate of infected cells, since the immune system can recognize viral proteins on the surface of infected cells and destroy them.

The distribution of HIV-infected cells in the body is determined primarily by the distribution of cells bearing CD4. The CD4 antigen was first identified by its presence on certain T cells, and indeed much of its normal function seems to involve assisting the complex network of communication among immune cells.

T cells bearing CD4 interact with cells known as antigen-presenting cells, which locate foreign antigens and display them on their own cell membrane, together with molecules known as Class II Major Histocompatibility Complex (MHC) glycoproteins. When helper T cells recognize this combination of an antigen and a Class II MHC glycoprotein, they initiate an immune response against other cells bearing the antigen, such as foreign or infected cells. It is thought that an interaction between CD4 antigens on the T cells and Class II MHC glycoproteins on the antigen-presenting cells is a crucial part of the encounter between the cells.

It is now known that T cells are not the only cells that have the CD4 antigen embedded in their membrane. As many as 40 percent of the peripheral-blood monocytes (cells that mature to become the scavenger cells known as macrophages), as well as certain antigen-presenting cells in the lymph nodes, skin and other organs, also express CD4 and can be infected by HIV. About 5 percent of the body's B cells (cells responsible for the production of antibodies) may also express CD4 and be susceptible to infection by HIV. In all these cells the presence of CD4 can be shown relatively easily.

On the other hand, in some other kinds of cells that can be infected by HIV in culture it is not possible to detect CD4 directly. These include certain cells of the brain known as glial cells, a range of malignant brain-tumor cells and some cell lines derived from cancers of the bowel. Nevertheless, although these cells do not produce detectable amounts of CD4, they do contain low levels of messenger RNA encoding the CD4 protein, indicating that they produce some CD4. Apparently the expression of only a very small amount of CD4 is sufficient for infection by HIV.

Cells of the gut also do not produce appreciable amounts of CD4, but Cecilia Cheng-Mayer and Levy at San Francisco have recently shown that the gut cells known as chromaffin cells do sometimes appear to be infected with HIV in vivo. They suggest that such a gut infection may be what leads to the AIDS-associated weight loss and emaciation known in Africa as Slim Disease. The role of CD4 in infections of brain cells and gut cells in vivo cannot be determined without further research. It is possible that in these cases the HIV particle binds to an alternative receptor molecule.

A number of workers have recently determined precisely which part of the CD4 molecule is the binding site for HIV. Most of the molecule lies outside the cell, but a small segment passes through the cell membrane and ends in a short intracellular "tail." The extracellular region consists of four domains that are similar in some ways to the "variable domains" of antibody molecules.

One way to determine the precise location of the binding site is to expose CD4 molecules to monoclonal antibodies that recognize various epitopes, or molecular shapes, on the CD4 molecule and note which antibodies block the binding of HIV to CD4. One group of antibodies, represented by the antibodies designated Leu3a and OKT4a, is particularly efficient at blocking the binding of HIV. Quentin J.

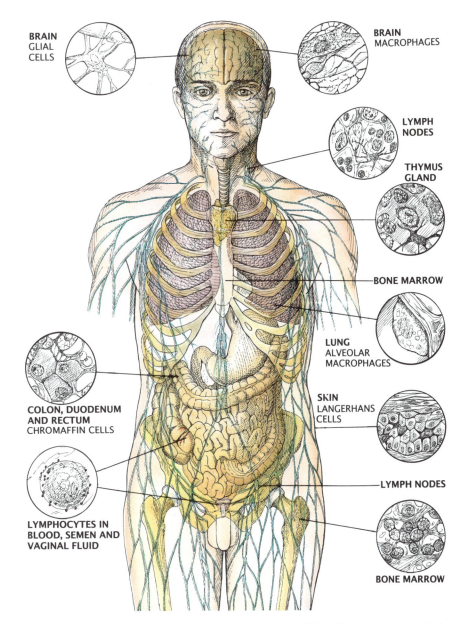

BRAIN
GLIAL
CELLS

BRAIN
MACROPHAGES

**LYMPH
NODES**

**THYMUS
GLAND**

BONE MARROW

**LUNG
ALVEOLAR
MACROPHAGES**

**COLON, DUODENUM
AND RECTUM**
CHROMAFFIN CELLS

**SKIN
LANGERHANS
CELLS**

LYMPH NODES

**LYMPHOCYTES IN
BLOOD, SEMEN AND
VAGINAL FLUID**

BONE MARROW

Figure 50 DISTRIBUTION OF TISSUES in the body that can be infected with HIV is closely linked to the distribution of cells bearing the CD4 molecule. With the possible exceptions of glial cells in the brain and chromaffin cells in the colon, duodenum and rectum, every cell that can be infected with HIV carries the CD4 molecule on its surface.

Sattentau and Peter C. L. Beverley of University College London have used large panels of anti-CD4 monoclonal antibodies to draw a "map" of the HIV binding site (that is, to determine which regions of the CD4 molecule are most important in binding HIV). They have found that the Leu3a antibody blocks not only HIV-1 and HIV-2 but also many strains of the simian immunodeficiency virus (SIV) (see Chapter 3, "The Origins of the AIDS Virus," by Max Essex and Phyllis J. Kanki). One implication of this finding is that the region of gp120 that is most important in binding to the cell is highly conserved, even among strains of virus whose envelope proteins are otherwise very different, having fewer than 40 percent of their amino acids (the basic building blocks of protein) in common. In another study, McClure and Sattentau have examined how

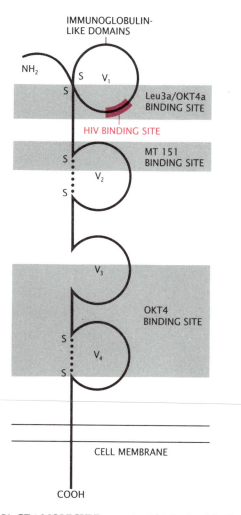

IMMUNOGLOBULIN-
LIKE DOMAINS

NH₂

S

S V₁

Leu3a/OKT4a
BINDING SITE

HIV BINDING SITE

MT 151
BINDING SITE

V₂

V₃

OKT4
BINDING SITE

V₄

CELL MEMBRANE

COOH

Figure 51 CD4 MOLECULE cannot yet be depicted in detail, but some features of its structure are known. Most of the molecule lies outside the cell, but a segment of it passes through the cell membrane and ends in a short tail inside the cell. Four sections of the molecule, designated V1, V2, V3 and V4, resemble the so-called variable domains of some immunoglobulin (antibody) molecules. The site to which the HIV gp120 molecule binds (color) lies in the outermost section. Shaded regions indicate areas in which binding sites of certain monoclonal antibodies (antibodies that recognize specific molecular configurations) lie. The so-called Leu3a/OKT4a group of monoclonal antibodies binds at the same site as HIV and can block infection by HIV.

well various epitopes of CD4 have been conserved during the course of evolution. They have demonstrated that the Leu3a monoclonal antibody reacts with all primate lymphocytes, including those of human beings, the great apes and African, Asian and New World monkeys, and prevents them from being infected in vitro with HIV. (In vivo most monkeys are not susceptible to HIV infection.) The implication is that the relevant parts of CD4 have been preserved even as the ancestors of these species diverged in other ways.

A further way to determine which parts of the CD4 and gp120 molecules are crucial for binding is to introduce deliberate mutations in the genes that encode the molecules. For example, an investigator might simply delete the genetic sequence that encodes a region of the CD4 molecule and test the resulting mutant's ability to bind HIV.

Early experiments, in which large sections of the CD4 molecule were deleted, indicated that the amino-terminal domain of the molecule (the section farthest from the cell membrane) is essential for the binding of gp120. Ned Landau and Littman at San Francisco have confirmed these results in experiments in which segments of mouse CD4 were combined with segments of human CD4. Mouse CD4 is broadly similar to the human molecule, but it is not recognized by gp120 or by the monoclonal antibodies that are specific to human CD4. The "chimeric" molecules do bind gp120 very well if the first 100 amino acids at the amino-terminal end of the molecule are human, even if the rest of the molecule is derived from the mouse. (The CD4 molecule as a whole consists of 433 amino acids.)

In experiments that were even more specific, Andrew Peterson and Brian Seed of the Harvard Medical School made hundreds of tiny "point mutations" in the human CD4 gene. They found that about seven amino acids residing near the middle of the initial 100-amino-acid segment are crucial for recognition by gp120 and by such monoclonal antibodies as Leu3a and OKT4a, which can block the binding of gp120. The major site on CD4 that is recognized by gp120, then, is a small region in the outermost part of the CD4 molecule.

The parts of gp120 that are essential for binding have also been analyzed by mutagenesis. William A. Haseltine's group at the Dana-Farber Cancer Institute and Larry Lasky's group at Genentech Inc. have shown that three distinct regions of gp120 are essential for the recognition and binding of CD4. Probably these regions come together to form a pocket that fits the binding site on CD4 when the gp120 molecule folds into its normal three-dimensional configuration.

Knowledge of the interactions through which HIV binds to target cells suggests several possible ways of blocking HIV infection. One method would be to inject subjects with so-called soluble CD4 molecules, which consist of segments of the portion of CD4 that normally lies outside the cell membrane. Soluble CD4 has been produced through recombinant-DNA technology by a number of laboratories and biotechnology companies. The molecules bind tightly to gp120; when they saturate all the gp120 on the virus's envelope, they neutralize its infectivity. Because the CD4-binding site on gp120 is essentially the same in all strains of

HIV and SIV, soluble CD4 can neutralize any strain of the virus, making it an attractive candidate for treatment.

Soluble CD4 would have some disadvantages as an AIDS therapy, however. First of all, it would have to be injected repeatedly in large doses. In addition, soluble CD4 might bind to Class II MHC glycoproteins, interfering with their normal function. That would exacerbate the immune deficiency of AIDS rather than curing it. The problem could be surmounted, however, if gp120 and the Class II MHC glycoproteins recognize different sites on CD4. It might then be possible to make smaller segments of the CD4 molecule that correspond just to the site recognized by gp120.

Another way to exploit our knowledge of the CD4 molecule involves molecules known as anti-

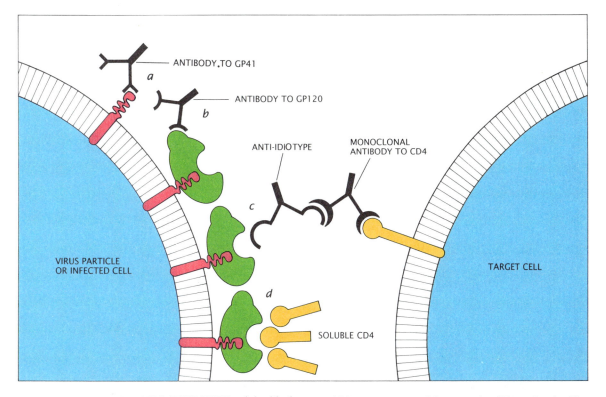

Figure 52 POTENTIAL AIDS THERAPIES might block the binding of the virus particle or an infected cell to a target cell. Among the simplest therapies are antibodies that bind to gp41 (a) or to gp120 (b). In another approach (c) the subject would be inoculated with monoclonal antibodies that bind to the CD4 molecule. The presence of these antibodies might stimulate the patient's immune system to produce "anti-idiotypes": a second set of antibodies, which would bear some resemblance to the CD4 molecule. The anti-idiotypes might bind to gp120 molecules, blocking them off and preventing them from binding to CD4 on target cells. Still another approach (d) would be to inject the subject with "soluble CD4" molecules (which consist of the portion of CD4 that normally lies outside the cell membrane). Soluble CD4 would bind tightly to gp120, blocking infection.

idiotype antibodies [see "Anti-idiotypes and Immunity," by Ronald C. Kennedy, Joseph L. Melnick and Gordon R. Dreesman; SCIENTIFIC AMERICAN, July, 1986]. A number of investigators, led by Ronald C. Kennedy and Gordon R. Dreesman of the Southwest Foundation for Biomedical Research in San Antonio, have inoculated mice with monoclonal antibodies that recognize the part of CD4 that is the binding site for gp120. These monoclonal antibodies are, in a sense, "negative images" of the binding site: they fit around the binding site on CD4 as a mitten fits a hand. In response to such an inoculation, the mouse immune system generates antibodies that bind to the monoclonal antibody. Some of these new antibodies, the so-called anti-idiotypes, fit precisely into the monoclonal antibody's CD4-binding site; they are new hands that fit inside the mitten.

In some cases the anti-idiotype has a shape very similar to that of the site on CD4 that is recognized by gp120. In a sense, then, these anti-idiotypes resemble CD4; like soluble CD4, they can bind to viral gp120 and should therefore be able to neutralize the infectivity of HIV.

Thus it may be possible to use anti-CD4 monoclonal antibodies as a kind of vaccine in human beings. In response to an injection of anti-CD4 monoclonal antibodies, the immune system might produce anti-idiotypes that bind to the virus and neutralize it. These anti-idiotypes would protect against all strains of the virus, because all strains of HIV recognize the same site on the CD4 molecule.

The actual neutralizing effect of such anti-idiotypes has been investigated independently by Dalgleish and by Sattentau and Beverley. They find that anti-idiotype antibodies do indeed neutralize HIV, but only very weakly. There are several possible explanations for such weak neutralization. First, it may be that the anti-idiotype antibody does not fit the gp120 protein very well. Second, the part of the gp120 molecule that recognizes CD4 probably resides in a pocket or crevice within the molecule, so that the relatively large antibodies cannot gain access to it easily. Third, the anti-idiotypes may not actually neutralize HIV at all; instead they may stimulate the immune system to produce another set of antibodies that have the opposite affinity: anti-anti-idiotypes, which might block the CD4 receptor just as the original antibody does.

People who are infected with HIV generate an impressive immune response to the virus. They produce antibodies to all the viral proteins, and their immune systems activate the various types of killer and scavenger cells that are part of any normal immune response. Yet once infection has occurred, these responses do not appear to halt the progress of the disease. Perhaps our increasing knowledge of the viral envelope and the cellular protein to which it binds will provide new approaches to defeating the virus.

AIDS Therapies

*One drug—AZT—is already in clinical use. New knowledge of HIV
makes it possible to design drugs that interrupt specific phases of
the viral life cycle. More effective therapies are on the way.*

• • •

Robert Yarchoan, Hiroaki Mitsuya and Samuel Broder

Back in 1984, when AIDS was conclusively shown to be caused by the human immuno-deficiency virus (HIV), many investigators and clinicians doubted that a drug capable of attacking the virus directly would ever be found. Their fears were understandable: past efforts to find antiviral drugs had turned up only a handful of effective agents. Moreover, retroviruses such as HIV present a particularly elusive target: they can integrate into the genome of body cells, where they can lie dormant and go undetected for long periods of time.

In the case of HIV, the problem is exacerbated by the virus's ability to infect a variety of tissues and cells in the body. In particular, the virus can hide in cells of the central nervous system, where it is protected by the blood-brain barrier, which many drugs cannot pierce. Even if certain drugs could cross the barrier, brain cells already damaged by the virus may never heal. Also, secondary diseases associated with AIDS, such as Kaposi's sarcoma, aggressive lymphomas and certain opportunistic infections, can lead to complications that may be difficult to eradicate in their own right. The complexity of HIV, combined with the devastating nature of the disease itself, led many to regard AIDS as a uniquely challenging and perhaps insurmountable problem.

That grim prognosis, however, has improved in a remarkably short time. A survey of off-the-shelf antiviral substances, initiated in our laboratory at the National Cancer Institute (NCI), turned up one, azidothymidine (AZT), that has already been shown to prolong the lives of certain AIDS patients. In the past four years investigators have come to understand the life cycle of the AIDS virus better than that of perhaps any other virus, and with that understanding we have begun to be able to rationally design drug therapies aimed at specific stages during which the virus might be vulnerable. We expect such drugs to have a major impact on this disease in the future.

Any therapeutic agent against an infection caused by a pathogen, whether it is a virus, bacteria, fungus or protozoan, must either kill the pathogen or stop it from multiplying. This it must do without harming the infected host significantly. Generally such drugs accomplish their task by attacking a biochemical pathway unique to the pathogen. In the case of bacteria this is relatively easy to do, because there are many differences between the

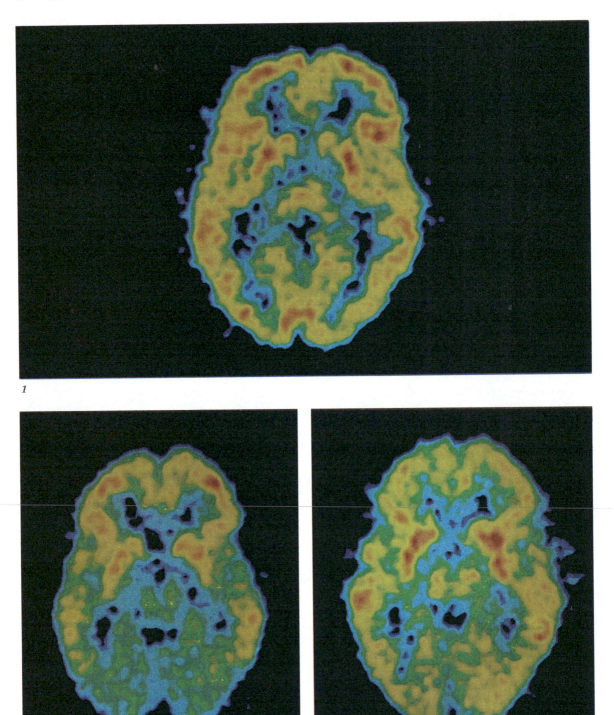

1

2

3

structure and metabolism of bacterial cells and those of mammalian cells. Penicillin, for example, interferes with the synthesis of bacterial cell walls; mammalian cells, because they lack these cell walls, are not affected by the drug.

Viruses present a more formidable problem. Viruses are simply packets of genetic material (RNA in the case of the AIDS virus) cloaked in glycoproteins and lipids. They cannot replicate on their own. Instead they infect cells of another organism and commandeer the cells' genetic machinery in order to reproduce. When viruses are actively replicating, it is often difficult to distinguish between viral proteins that interact with the cell and host-cell proteins themselves. The host cells' intimate involvement in many stages of the life cycle of the virus makes it difficult to find agents that selectively inhibit viral replication while damaging the host as little as possible.

Moreover, virtually no drug—not even penicillin—is completely devoid of side effects and toxicity. One must therefore always consider the balance between harm to the pathogen and harm to the host. An essential aspect of any potential drug is its "therapeutic index": the ratio of the toxic dose to the effective dose. Drugs to treat a minor illness must have a high therapeutic index. For a life-threatening illness such as AIDS, one may have to accept drugs with a lower therapeutic index, at least in the beginning.

Against this background one can begin to appreciate some of the considerations surrounding the search for AIDS therapies. In the summer of 1984 two of us (Mitsuya and Broder) obtained the AIDS virus from Robert C. Gallo's group and began testing a number of substances for activity against HIV. Many of these had previously been shown to be active against mouse retroviruses by a number of investigators, including Wolfram Ostertag of the

Max Planck Institute for Experimental Medicine in Göttingen, Philip Furmanski of the Michigan Cancer Foundation, Joel A. Huberman of the Roswell Park Memorial Institution and Eric De Clercq of the Rega Institute in Leuven, Belgium. Their work had languished in relative obscurity for years because no pathogenic human retroviruses had yet been identified—and in any case many people assumed that retroviral infections were by their very nature untreatable. The urgent search for a drug against AIDS revived our interest in this earlier work. By the late spring of 1985, 15 of the 300 drugs tested had been found to stop HIV replication in the test tube.

One of these was 3'-azido-2',3'-dideoxythymidine, or AZT (also called azidothymidine or zidovudine). We began an intensive effort to develop AZT as a drug suitable for the therapy of AIDS. We gave the drug to the first patient on July 3, 1985. By the end of that year our group, in collaboration with workers at Duke University and the Wellcome Research Laboratories in Durham, N.C., could infer that AZT was active in some HIV-infected patients. By September, 1986, clinical studies at 12 U.S. medical centers demonstrated that AZT can improve both the survival period and the quality of life for patients with AIDS. For the first time, a drug was shown to exert a positive effect against a pathogenic retroviral infection. An intensive global effort is now under way to find other agents for the treatment of AIDS.

To understand how these agents might work, one must consider the structure and replicative cycle of the AIDS virus. In HIV and other retroviruses, genetic information flows in a backward, or "retro," direction: from RNA to DNA, whereas the usual direction for other organisms is from DNA to RNA. Retroviruses achieve this feat by means of a special enzyme, reverse transcriptase, which can take RNA and exploit it as a template for assembling a corresponding strand of DNA.

Replication in HIV is a complicated affair involving a large number of steps. The virus's outer coat of glycoprotein binds and fuses to the membrane of a host cell, enabling the viral RNA, along with reverse transcriptase, to invade the cell's cytoplasm. There the reverse transcriptase synthesizes DNA from the viral RNA; the DNA then inserts itself into the host's chromosomes. Later this "proviral" DNA may be transcribed back to RNA, which the cell's protein-production machinery translates into viral proteins. These proteins reassemble into complete

Figure 53 THREE BRAIN SCANS reveal that HIV-induced dementia can be relieved by treatment with azidothymidine (AZT). Red and yellow regions correspond to areas of high metabolic activity. Scan 1 is that of a healthy individual. Scan 2 is from a patient with dementia caused by HIV infection; it shows relatively reduced activity in several brain regions. Scan 3 is from the same patient after treatment with AZT. Metabolic activity became closer to normal. The patient's intellectual function also improved. (Positron emission tomography scans by S. M. Larson, G. Berg and A. Brunetti of the Clinical Center of the National Institutes of Health. The Wellcome Research Laboratories supplied the AZT used in all our studies.)

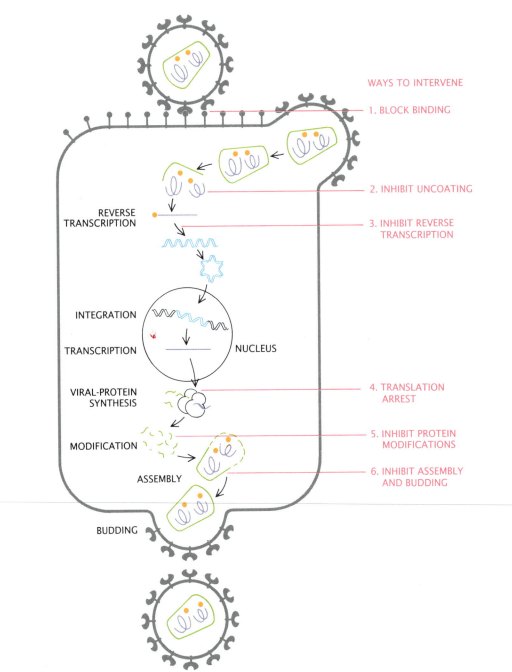

WAYS TO INTERVENE

1. BLOCK BINDING

2. INHIBIT UNCOATING

REVERSE
TRANSCRIPTION

3. INHIBIT REVERSE
TRANSCRIPTION

INTEGRATION

TRANSCRIPTION   NUCLEUS

VIRAL-PROTEIN
SYNTHESIS

4. TRANSLATION
ARREST

MODIFICATION

5. INHIBIT PROTEIN
MODIFICATIONS

ASSEMBLY

6. INHIBIT ASSEMBLY
AND BUDDING

BUDDING

Figure 54 HIV LIFE CYCLE is subject to attack by drugs at several stages. Certain antibodies could block the binding of the viral envelope glycoprotein, gp120, to CD4 receptors on the surface of helper *T* cells (*1*). Other agents might keep viral RNA and reverse transcriptase from escaping their protein coat (*2*). Drugs such as AZT and other dideoxynucleosides prevent the reverse transcription of viral RNA into viral DNA (*3*). Later on, antisense oligonucleotides could block the translation of mRNA into viral proteins (*4*). Before they can be assembled, viral proteins must be modified; certain compounds could interfere with such processes as the cleavage of proteins or the addition of sugar groups (*5*). Finally, such antiviral substances as interferons could keep the virus particle from assembling itself and budding out of the cell (*6*).

virus particles, which emerge from the host cell and can infect new cells. It is clear that HIV's complex life cycle helps the virus to infect—and evade—cells of the immune system. From the therapist's standpoint this complexity may prove to be as much a boon as it is a curse: it provides many targets for antiviral agents to attack during the life cycle of HIV.

The first stage at which an anti-HIV agent might intervene is during the binding of the virus to a cell. HIV has an envelope glycoprotein called gp120, which forms a strong bond with a glycoprotein called CD4 (or T4), found on the surface of certain cells in the body. CD4 is particularly abundant on the surface of a class of white blood cells called helper T cells, which are therefore a prime target for HIV infection. Indeed, a gradual depletion of such cells is a hallmark of AIDS. Normally helper T cells are crucial regulators of immune defense systems. Without enough functioning helper T cells, infected individuals become subject to opportunistic infections and malignancies.

HIV-infected helper T cells do not work as well as they should, and they can be killed outright by the virus. In addition, studies in test tubes have shown that a few infected cells can kill large numbers of uninfected cells through a process called syncytium formation: the fusion of an infected cell with healthy cells. Jeffrey D. Lifson and Edgar G. Engleman of Stanford University, William A. Haseltine of the Dana-Farber Cancer Institute and their colleagues showed that syncytia are initiated when the gp120 on virus particles at the surface of infected cells binds to CD4 on the surface of healthy cells. A drug that interferes with viral binding therefore may not only interrupt the viral life cycle but also block the formation of syncytia.

There are several approaches to inhibiting the initial binding of HIV to a cell. One approach is to develop an antibody that binds to a critical part of the viral envelope, thereby neutralizing the gp120's ability to bind to CD4. Such an antibody could be linked to a toxin; it could then bind to and destroy infected cells, such as macrophages, that harbor the virus and produce HIV proteins. One might also develop antibodies to CD4, but such an approach is potentially hazardous, because the antibodies would attack the body's healthy immune cells. Most research, therefore, has focused on antibodies to gp120.

There are inherent difficulties in creating an ef-fective neutralizing antibody to gp120. Not all antibodies to gp120 will block the critical CD4-binding site. Moreover, patients who produce neutralizing antibodies (generally only in low concentrations) as a natural response to HIV infection may still develop AIDS. Why is that? No one is certain, but one reason may be that HIV has a high rate of mutation. Some variants may have an altered envelope glycoprotein that cannot be neutralized by the antibodies. A second reason may be that sugar chains on the envelope glycoprotein are similar to those on the surface of human cells, so that the envelope lacks enough unique sites to which an antibody can bind. A third reason may be that the CD4-binding site is in a deep cleft in the envelope glycoprotein, making it relatively inaccessible. Finally, it is possible that the crucial sites are exposed only during binding and are hidden from the immune system most of the time.

In order to overcome these difficulties, investigators have tried several approaches. One is to develop a monoclonal antibody by identifying an antibody that does bind to a critical site, and then to clone it and grow it in the test tube. With this method, Shuzo Matsushita of Kumamoto University and his colleagues recently produced a neutralizing antibody to gp120 that they call $0.5\text{-}\beta$. This antibody neutralizes some, but not all, strains of HIV. A similar approach may in the future produce antibodies to a broader range of HIV strains.

A second approach is to make an "anti-idiotypic antibody": an antibody to an antibody against CD4. The idea is that a monoclonal antibody against CD4 might resemble the CD4-binding site on gp120, and therefore an antibody (the anti-idiotype) made against this anti-CD4 antibody (the idiotype) might in turn bind to gp120. The concept is somewhat analogous to making a negative from a photographic negative to produce a positive. To investigate this possibility, two groups, one led by Ronald C. Kennedy of the Southwest Foundation for Biomedical Research and the other by Peter C. L. Beverley of University College London, took several CD4 antibodies known to inhibit HIV binding and produced several monoclonal antibodies to them. Both groups found that some of these anti-idiotypic antibodies bound to and neutralized HIV in vitro.

Another approach is to create a free-floating, or soluble, form of CD4 that can bind to HIV, monopolizing its CD4-binding sites and thus keeping it from binding to the CD4 on a helper T cell. Soluble

CD4 was recently produced with recombinant-DNA methods by five groups, including researchers at Genentech Inc., Biogen N.V., Columbia University, the Smith Kline & French Laboratories, the Dana-Farber Cancer Institute and the Basel Institute for Immunology. These molecules did indeed adhere to the CD4-binding sites on the HIV envelope and inhibit the virus from infecting T cells. It will probably be difficult for the virus to mutate in such a way that it loses its affinity for the CD4 molecule while retaining its ability to infect T cells. We plan to

begin testing the substance (called rCD4) in AIDS patients in the very near future.

In the future it may be possible to create "chimeric" molecules by taking the sites on CD4 that bind to HIV and splicing them onto the constant part of a human immunoglobulin (antibody) molecule. There are several possible advantages to such "customized antibodies." We think certain parts of the so-called heavy chain of the immunoglobulin molecule may be able to activate other parts of the immune system into destroying the virus. The chi-

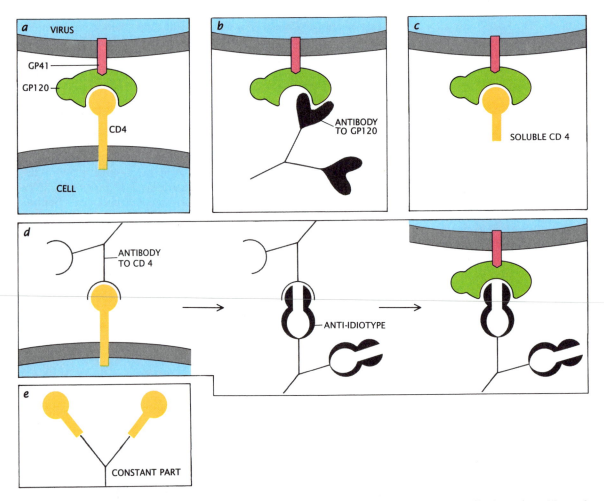

Figure 55 VIRAL BINDING depends on the interaction of viral envelope glycoprotein, gp120 (*green*), with CD4 receptors (*yellow*) on the surface of helper T cells (*a*). An antibody directed against gp120 could block the site that binds to CD4 (*b*); so could a soluble form of the CD4 protein (*c*). An "anti-idiotypic antibody" (*d*) to gp120 is made by taking a monoclonal antibody against CD4 and forming an antibody to it. A "chimeric" molecule (*e*) could be more stable than soluble CD4; it combines gp120-binding sites on the CD4 molecule with the constant region of an immunoglobulin molecule.

meric molecule would act like a bloodhound-and-policeman team: the CD4 sniffs out the virus, and the immunoglobulin radios for the troops. What is more, the chimeric molecule may stay in circulation for a longer time than soluble CD4 alone, because certain immunoglobulins have a long half-life in the bloodstream. Such an approach has never been tried in human beings, but structural similarities between CD4 and immunoglobulins (CD4 belongs to the immunoglobulin "supergene" family) give us hope that such chimeras will retain functional properties of both molecules.

The approaches described above involve complex biological molecules that bind to HIV envelope glycoprotein. Other molecules, however, may also do the trick. Several large, sulfated, negatively charged molecules have been shown to inhibit HIV replication. One prototype is dextran sulfate. Molecules weighing between 7,000 and 8,000 daltons inhibit HIV replication in vitro, as recently shown by Ryuji Ueno and Sachiko Kuno of Ueno Fine Chemicals Industry, Ltd., in Osaka, Japan, Masahiko Ito of Fukushima Medical College and two of us (Mitsuya and Broder) at the NCI. Our group found that one way this compound may have its effect is by inhibiting viral binding. Dextran sulfate has also been shown to inhibit syncytia formation in vitro, as one

would expect from a molecule that blocks viral binding.

Dextran sulfates have been administered for some time as plasma expanders, anticoagulants and cholesterol-lowering drugs. This clinical history suggests (but by no means proves) that the anti-HIV form of dextran sulfate may be relatively nontoxic. It remains to be seen, however, whether doses sufficient to inhibit HIV can be achieved by giving the drug orally, or indeed whether it will be effective at all against AIDS. Also, we do not yet know whether the drug will interact with other drugs in patients. Donald I. Abrams is studying dextran sulfate in patients at the San Francisco General Hospital.

After HIV has bound to a cell, it fuses with the cell membrane, releasing its contents into the cytoplasm. There the inner protein coat is partially removed to expose the viral RNA. Antibodies could neutralize gp41, the envelope glycoprotein that mediates fusion, and so prevent fusion from occurring. Antiviral drugs may be able to interfere with the uncoating process.

The target that has received perhaps more attention than any other, however, is the next stage of viral replication: the synthesis of viral DNA by the enzyme reverse transcriptase. This strategy is attrac-

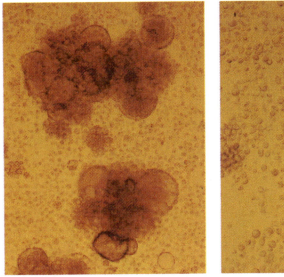
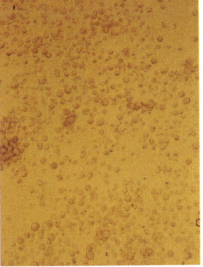

Figure 56 SYNCYTIA are giant, multinucleated structures that form when HIV-infected cells fuse with uninfected cells, as is seen in this phase-contrast micrograph (*left*). They occur because viral envelope glycoprotein on the surface of infected cells binds to CD4 molecules on other cells. Dextran sulfate, which may inhibit viral binding, prevents syncytium formation in a mixed culture of infected and uninfected cells (*right*).

tive because it attacks a step that is unique to retro-viruses. Early in our own efforts to find an anti-retroviral agent, we made this our prime target. In particular we focused on compounds belonging to a family of reverse-transcriptase inhibitors called di-deoxynucleosides. These are nucleoside analogues, molecules that closely resemble the nucleotides that serve as building blocks in DNA and RNA: the pyrimidines (thymidine, uridine and cytidine) and the purines (adenosine and guanosine).

One such compound is 3'-azido-2', 3'-dideoxy-thymidine, the AZT we mentioned above. AZT was originally synthesized in 1964 by Jerome P. Horwitz of the Michigan Cancer Foundation as a potential anticancer drug . (It failed, but Burroughs Wellcome continued to make it). In February, 1985, our labo-ratory found it to be a potent inhibitor of HIV in T-cell cultures at concentrations of between one and five micromolar (or between about .25 and 1.25 micrograms per milliliter). Moreover, the compound was not significantly toxic to T cells below concen-trations of from 20 to 50 micromolar. Soon after this work, AZT proved to be effective in AIDS patients at concentrations of between one and five micromolar, the amount initially predicted by our T-cell assay system.

How does AZT protect T cells against HIV? The key lies in its resemblance to the nucleoside thymidine. In the cell, enzymes add phosphate groups (in a process called phosphorylation) to con-vert AZT into AZT triphosphate, the active form of the drug. (AZT triphosphate cannot be given di-rectly because cells cannot absorb it.) AZT triphos-phate is an analogue of thymidine triphosphate, one of the building blocks of DNA, and it appears to inhibit the production of viral DNA by at least two mechanisms: competitive inhibition and chain termination.

In competitive inhibition, AZT triphosphate binds to reverse transcriptase at a site that ordinarily binds to physiological nucleoside triphosphates. In chain termination, reverse transcriptase is fooled into in-corporating AZT triphosphate in a growing chain of viral DNA in place of the normal thymidine tri-phosphate. When it tries to add the next link, it is thwarted because AZT triphosphate lacks the hy-droxyl (OH) group that is needed to forge the chem-ical bond to the next link. The virus cannot repair this mistake, and the viral DNA synthesis comes grinding to a halt.

Other dideoxynucleosides that are active against HIV also appear to work by these mechanisms. All these compounds appear to be effective against a number of retroviruses (indeed, against every one tested so far), but only when they are in the triphos-phate form. Their therapeutic effectiveness, then, depends in part on how easily they enter cells and undergo phosphorylation by cellular enzymes called kinases. This process is in fact more efficient for some compounds than it is for others. For exam-ple, 2',3'-dideoxythymidine—which is AZT with a hydrogen atom in place of the azido (N_3) group—is poorly phosphorylated in human cells and so is less potent than AZT against HIV. In addition, the way these compounds are phosphorylated varies greatly among different species. Animal models, therefore, may not accurately predict whether a particular di-deoxynucleoside will be effective in human beings.

Another question is whether mutation might alter the viral reverse transcriptase so that it is no longer inhibited by AZT. This is not idle speculation: it happens that AZT works because the virus's reverse transcriptase actually prefers AZT triphosphate, and tends to bind and incorporate it rather than thymi-dine triphosphate. The DNA polymerases in mam-malian cells, however, do not prefer AZT triphos-phate, and so the host cell can continue to function. Reverse transcriptase might be altered in such a way that it too will not prefer AZT triphosphate.

In an attempt to study this point, Brendan A. Larder, Graham K. Darby and their colleagues at the Wellcome Research Laboratories in the U.K. mu-tated HIV reverse transcriptase in specific ways. They found that some of the altered reverse tran-scriptases were more resistant to inhibition by AZT triphosphate. These agents were, however, im-paired in their normal activity. No one knows whether viruses with such mutations would be in-fectious or cause disease; specifically, no one is sure whether AZT-resistant mutants can arise in pa-tients.

Another point to consider with dideoxynucleo-sides is that because they resemble important cellu-lar chemicals, they may interact with a variety of enzymes in the body. For example, 2',3'-dideoxy-adenosine (ddA) in triphosphate form is a potent HIV inhibitor in vitro, but in the body ddA is more likely to be converted by the ubiquitous enzyme adenosine deaminase into 2',3'-dideoxyinosine (ddI), which in its phosphorylated form is only weakly active against HIV. Yet ddI is effective against HIV in culture because it is itself metabo-lized to ddA triphosphate in cells. In fact this may

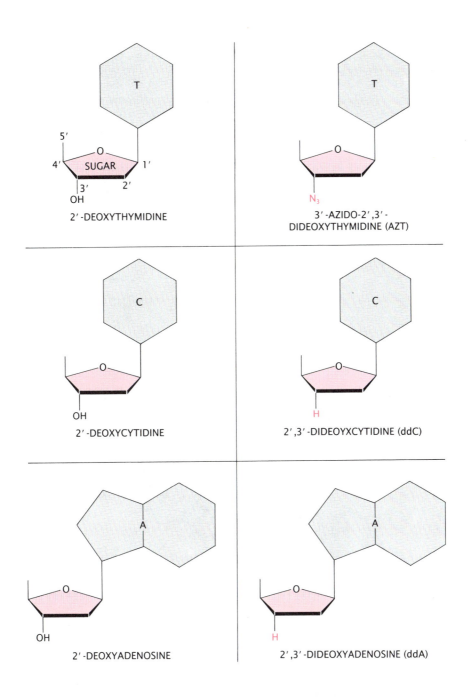

Figure 57 DIDEOXYNUCLEOSIDE ANALOGUES (*right column*) could prove to be potent drugs against HIV because of their resemblance to deoxynucleosides (*left column*), the building blocks of DNA. Both types of molecules consist of a base—here thymine (*T*), cytosine (*C*) or adenine (*A*)—joined to a sugar ring. A hydroxyl group (OH) on the sugar ring forms a bond that links one nucleotide to another in a DNA chain. In the analogues the hydroxyl group is replaced by a group that is unable to form the link.

be the dominant pathway by which ddA is phosphorylated in the body. We may not be as lucky with other compounds, however, which might simply be converted into useless metabolites before they can reach target cells.

After a strand of DNA has been copied from the viral RNA, the reverse transcription proceeds to a second stage: the synthesis of a second DNA copy of the first DNA strand. This stage is also subject to attack. One could, for example, try to interfere with the viral enzyme RNase H, which chops up viral RNA in an orderly fashion after the first DNA copy of it has been made, thus making room for the second DNA strand. It may also be possible to block another enzyme, viral integrase,

which is thought to serve as a chemical sewing kit that cuts the DNA of the host cell before stitching viral DNA into the site of the cut.

The next target for therapy presents itself some time later in the cycle of HIV, when the host cell is activated. The cell may begin to produce new proteins or receptors, and it may divide. The same process that activates the cell may also trigger the transcription and translation of viral DNA into viral proteins. We and others are investigating whether this process can be interrupted by the use of "antisense oligonucleotides," an approach first suggested more than 15 years ago by Paul C. Zamecnik of the Worcester Foundation for Experimental Biology. The idea is to create short nucleotide sequences, or oligonucleotides, that are complementary to a part

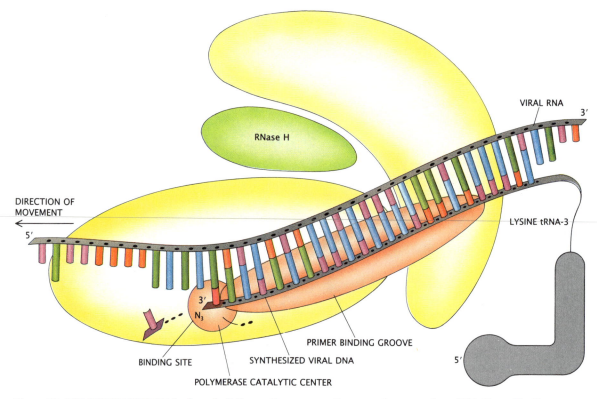

Figure 58 AZT TRIPHOSPHATE (*red*) can halt the synthesis of viral DNA. Reverse transcriptase (*yellow*) binds to viral RNA and to a lysine tRNA-3, which provides the starting point for the DNA. The growing strand sits in the primer binding groove. After the DNA strand is completed, RNase H removes the RNA so that a second DNA strand can form in its place. Cellular enzymes add three phosphates (*black dots*) to nucleosides such as thymidine, **as well as to analogues such as AZT. Normally, the reverse transcriptase then cleaves off two of the phosphates, and the remaining phosphate forms a phosphodiester linkage to the hydroxyl group at the end of the chain. But if AZT triphosphate is added instead, no further nucleotides can be added because the azido (N_3) group of AZT cannot form the linkage, and so viral DNA synthesis stops.**

of the viral mRNA. (The mRNA is in the "sense" mode, that is, it directly codes for proteins; these oligonucleotides are "antisense," that is, complementary to the mRNA.) These antisense constructs can bind to viral mRNA sequences in a process called hybridization, possibly obstructing the cell's ribosomes from moving along the RNA and thereby halting the translation of RNA into viral protein. This is called translation arrest or ribosomal-hybridization arrest.

One disadvantage with oligonucleotides is that many of them can be degraded by enzymes in the host cells. They can, however, be made resistant by modifying certain phosphate links between the nucleotides. For example, one can substitute a sulfur atom for one of the oxygen atoms to form a phosphorothioate. Makoto Matsukura in our group, working with Gerald Zon of Applied Biosystems, Inc., and Jack C. Cohen and Cy A. Stein of the NCI, recently found that such antisense phosphorothioates can indeed inhibit HIV production in cells chronically infected by HIV.

It may also be possible to stop viral production by blocking viral genes or proteins that regulate this process. The translation of viral RNA into protein is tightly controlled by the virus. Regulatory sequences, called long terminal repeats, at each end of the viral genome may directly control viral protein synthesis. Several viral proteins regulate this process as well. These regions might provide targets for selectively inhibiting HIV replication.

In addition, HIV replication can be influenced by proteins made by the host cell or even by other viruses that happen to also infect the cell. Gary J. Nabel and David Baltimore of the Whitehead Institute for Biomedical Research have recently shown that the cellular protein NF-κB, which acts as an intracellular activation signal in certain lymphocytes, may turn on HIV replication. Certain herpes viruses produce a protein called ICPO that can also trigger HIV replication. In patients infected with both a herpes virus and HIV, it may therefore be possible to delay the progress of AIDS by controlling the herpes infection, for example with the drug acyclovir.

After the viral proteins are produced, they undergo a series of modifications that result in a complete, functional virus. In one of these steps a viral enzyme cleaves the viral proteins. Because this enzyme is unique to HIV, several laboratories are now searching for agents that specifically inhibit it. In another step viral proteins gain carbohydrates in a

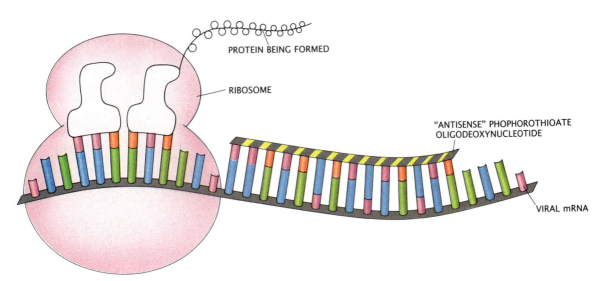

Figure 59 ANTISENSE OLIGONUCLEOTIDES are segments of DNA that are complementary to a portion of HIV mRNA. They are thought to bind to the viral mRNA and so prevent ribosomes from translating the mRNA into viral proteins. Oligonucleotides, however, are rapidly degraded by cellular enzymes. To make them resistant to the enzymes, one can substitute a sulfur atom (*yellow*) for an oxygen on the phosphate links between the nucleotides. The resulting compound, which is called a phosphorothioate, is resistant to degradation and has been shown to inhibit the expression of HIV in vitro.

process called glycosylation, in which enzymes add sugars and then other enzymes called trimming glycosidases trim off some of the terminal sugar groups. Two teams, one led by Joseph G. Sodroski and Haseltine and the other led by Robert Gruter of the Netherlands Red Cross Transfusion Service, recently showed that when HIV is produced in the presence of castanospermine, a plant alkaloid that inhibits a trimming glycosidase, it is less able to form syncytia or to infect cells. Castanospermine analogues, designed to be more potent and yet less toxic than castanospermine itself, might provide a treatment for HIV infection.

Finally, the viral proteins and RNA are transported to the cell membrane and there assembled into virus particles, which escape by budding out of the cell surface. The budding may be stopped by interferons, antiviral substances that are produced naturally in cells. Interferons are thought to act at other steps in the HIV life cycle as well. Certain substances that can induce a cell to produce interferon have also been found to inhibit HIV replication in vitro. Indeed, interferons have a wide range of effects and therefore may benefit AIDS patients in several ways. For example, alpha-interferon helps to suppress Kaposi's sarcoma, and so it might benefit certain AIDS patients by acting as both an anti-retroviral and an antitumor agent.

Of all the substances that show activity against HIV, AZT has undergone the most extensive clinical study. Five months after our laboratory showed in February of 1985 that AZT inhibits HIV replication, we administered the drug to the first patient in the Clinical Center at the National Institutes of Health (NIH). This patient had AIDS and had recently recovered from Pneumocystis carinii pneumonia. His immune functions were severely suppressed and his helper T cells were markedly depleted. When we exposed his skin to common antigens (in a test analogous to a tuberculosis test), he failed to produce the reddish swelling that signals a normal immune reaction. After taking AZT for several weeks, he gained weight and had an increased number of helper T cells. He also reacted to the skin test, indicating that the overall function of his T-cell immune system had improved.

Other patients at the NIH and at the Duke University Medical Center who received AZT in this first trial also had improved clinical symptoms and immunological function, which we attributed to the drug's antiviral effect. We also found that AZT could reduce the amount of HIV present in patients. In many cases, however, these improvements were only temporary, and, given the side effects that occurred in some patients, some investigators questioned whether the benefits were sufficient to have a substantial impact on the course of the disease.

To find out, the Wellcome group organized a randomized, placebo-controlled trial of AZT in 12 major medical centers around the U.S. Margaret A. Fischl of the University of Miami, Douglas D. Richman of the University of California at San Diego and their colleagues studied some 280 patients. These patients had either recovered from Pneumocystis carinii pneumonia or had severe AIDS-related complex. They were randomly chosen to receive either AZT or a placebo. Neither doctor nor patient knew whether the patient was receiving AZT or the placebo. Patients were not given any prophylaxis for the pneumonia, nor were they given any other AIDS therapy.

Six months into the trial, 19 patients in the placebo group had died, whereas only one patient in the group receiving AZT had died. Also, patients receiving AZT had fewer complications of the disease. At this point the trial was halted and all the patients were offered AZT. It now appears that AZT can increase the median survival time of patients with advanced AIDS by about a year. (The median survival time is the time at which 50 percent of the patients have died.) This evidence prompted the Food and Drug Administration, in March of 1987, to approve AZT as a prescription drug for severe HIV infection.

AZT may have an even greater effect if it is given earlier in the course of HIV infection. In fact, it is possible that it may actually prevent the progress of AIDS in at least some individuals, perhaps both by its direct antiviral effect and by partially restoring immune function. Gene M. Shearer of the NCI and Robert T. Schooley and Martin S. Hirsch of the Massachusetts General Hospital have shown that T cells from patients given AZT may be better able to kill HIV-infected cells. Clinical trials are now under way to test this idea. We wish to stress that until these trials are concluded, it will not be possible to draw valid inferences about the role of AZT in the early stages of HIV infection. Moreover, the long-term toxicity of AZT is not yet known.

Our early work with AZT showed it could penetrate into the fluid surrounding the brain, and so we wondered if it could treat the devastating dementia that sometimes develops in patients infected with HIV. When we gave AZT to afflicted patients, in most cases in which careful tests of intellectual function were done we found at least temporary improvement. This was apparent within the first few weeks of therapy. In addition, Philip A. Pizzo of the Pediatric Branch of the NCI has given continuous infusions of AZT to a number of children with AIDS, whose intelligence quotient (IQ) had fallen as a result of the disease. In some cases he found that the IQ returned to normal levels during treatment. (See Figure 53.)

We do not understand all the mechanisms that lead to AIDS dementia, and so the beneficial mechanisms of AZT are also unclear. It is of course possible that the improvements directly result from controlling HIV infection in the brain. Carlo-Federico Perno in our group has shown that cells of the monocyte-macrophage lineage, prime targets for HIV infection in the nervous system, can be protected against HIV replication even by low concentrations of AZT and other dideoxynucleosides. Whether this accounts for the clinical improvement in these patients, or whether another mechanism is involved, is a matter for further research.

Because of the rapid development of AZT, there remain many unanswered questions regarding its effects and the best method of administration. We do not know if it is better to keep AZT circulating at as constant a level as possible or to allow it to fluctuate. AZT levels decline by about 50 percent over the course of one hour, and the present schedule of one dose every four hours is designed to keep circulating levels fairly constant. In the case of dideoxynucleosides, one must also consider the metabolism of the phosphorylated products. For example, David G. Johns of the NCI has found that the intracellular half-life of ddA triphosphate, a metabolite of both ddA and its alter ego ddI, may be as high as 24 hours. It may therefore be possible to give ddA to patients just once or twice a day.

In spite of its beneficial effects, AZT is not a final answer. The drug can be toxic, particularly to bone marrow, so that patients on AZT often develop anemia (a decrease in red blood cells) and in some instances low numbers of white blood cells and platelets as well. Indeed, this often limits the amount of AZT that can be administered, particularly in patients with established AIDS, and bone-marrow suppression is a major reason for failure of the drug. The mechanism of toxicity remains unclear at present, but there is some evidence that it may not necessarily occur with other dideoxynucleosides.

Ultimately, the only way to tell whether other dideoxynucleosides that display anti-HIV activity in tissue culture will be more beneficial than AZT is to test them in patients. To this end, our group at the NCI and a multicenter group headed by Thomas C. Merigan, Jr., of the Stanford University School of Medicine recently conducted clinical trials of 2',3'-dideoxycytidine (ddC) in patients suffering from severe HIV infection. These studies showed that ddC can markedly reduce the amount of HIV replication and can also induce some improvements in immune function. Unfortunately patients who took continuous high doses of ddC for more than from eight to 12 weeks developed a painful peripheral neuropathy (a disorder of peripheral sensory and motor nerves), primarily in the feet. This neuropathy gradually subsided after patients stopped taking the drug.

Because the toxicity of ddC is different from that of AZT, we wondered whether we could obtain a better result if the two drugs were alternated. Such a regimen might allow vulnerable tissues to recover from the toxic effects of each drug; similar strategies have been successful in treating and even curing certain cancers. Some patients are now on an alternating regimen of ddC and AZT. Preliminary results show that some patients can tolerate such a treatment for more than a year without developing either neuropathy or suppressed bone marrow.

The dideoxynucleoside ddA and its metabolite ddI also strongly inhibit HIV in culture. These drugs appear to be less toxic in cultures of helper T cells than either AZT or ddC. In addition they are less toxic to bone marrow in culture. We are now carrying out trials to determine the toxicity and effective dose of ddA and ddI in patients. The preliminary results are encouraging.

The question posed at the beginning of this article has been answered in the affirmative. An antiretroviral drug, AZT, has been found that can reduce the severity of illness and prolong the survival of AIDS patients. AZT represents only a beginning, however, and it is certainly not a cure. Indeed, over time the true value of AZT may prove to be its validation of the key assumptions that underlie antiviral strategies for intervening in this illness.

In the future, as we learn more about how to attack HIV at different points in its life cycle, it may be possible to model AIDS therapies on successful

DRUG	MECHANISM OF ACTION	COMMENTS
DEXTRAN SULFATE	Probably inhibits viral binding	Used orally outside the U.S. to reduce cholesterol levels; prototype for polyanionic polysaccharides that have anti-HIV activity; Phase II clinical trials begun at San Francisco General Hospital.
SOLUBLE CD4 (ALSO CALLED rCD4)	Inhibits viral binding	Genetically engineered form of CD4; Phase I trials under way.
AZT (AZIDOTHYMIDINE OR ZIDOVUDINE)	Reverse-transcriptase inhibitor, chain terminator	Prescription drug; increases survival time and reduces opportunistic infections; can ameliorate HIV-induced dementia; toxic to bone marrow.
ddC	Reverse-transcriptase inhibitor, chain terminator	Antiviral effect even at very low dose; toxic effects on peripheral nerves can be reduced by taking alternately with AZT; Phase II trials under way both alone and in combination with AZT.
ddA and ddI	Reverse-transcriptase inhibitor, chain terminator	Relatively little bone-marrow toxicity in vitro; Phase I trials under way.
PHOSPHONOFORMATE	Reverse-transcriptase inhibitor	Also active against cytomegalovirus; Phase II trials show evidence of some activity against HIV.
RIFABUTIN	Possible reverse-transcriptase inhibitor	Also active in vitro against certain mycobacteria that can infect AIDS patients; Phase I trial being completed.
RIBAVIRAN	Mechanism unknown	Only partial anti-HIV effect; antagonizes activity of AZT in laboratory; clinical trials have so far not shown that it reduces HIV antigen in serum of patients.
PHOSPHOROTHIOATE OLIGODEOXYNUCLEOTIDES	Probably several mechanisms, including arrest of viral protein synthesis	May have sequence-specific and nonspecific activity; still in very early development.
CASTANOSPERMINE	Inhibits enzymes that trim sugar groups from viral proteins	Reduces syncytium formation and infectivity of virus; still in very early development.
ALPHA INTERFERON	May reduce viral budding; probably has other mechanisms as well	Also has direct antitumor activity against Kaposi's sarcoma; Phase II trials under way, both alone and in combination with AZT.
AMPLIGEN	Interferon inducer; may work by other mechanisms as well	Little toxicity observed in patients; large-scale Phase II and Phase III trials under way.

Figure 60 AIDS THERAPIES at various stages of testing are shown in this chart. All of the substances on the list have shown some activity against HIV in the test tube. Many of them are now in various stages of clinical trials. Phase I trials usually involve a small number of patients and are designed to establish toxicity, maximum tolerated dose and the drug's mechanism of action in the body. Phase II and Phase III trials involve larger numbers of people and are designed to assess the effectiveness of the drug.

therapies for cancers such as certain childhood leukemias. For example, as researchers develop agents that have different modes of activity against HIV, it may be possible to design multiple-drug therapies that will achieve better results than any one drug alone. In fact, investigators have already found that each of several drugs, including acyclovir (an antiherpes drug), ampligen, alpha-interferon and dextran sulfate, appears to have more than an additive effect when it is tested in vitro with AZT.

As with the treatment of childhood leukemia, it may be necessary to employ several phases of therapy. For example, one might first have to administer relatively toxic drugs that would halt viral replication and perhaps also destroy infected cells. One might then follow up with treatments that are capable of seeking out and suppressing hidden pockets of infection. Finally, the patient might be maintained on a low-dose regimen to suppress any recurrences. The drugs, the dosage and the dispensing schedule may differ from one phase to another. For example, a potent drug that might play a crucial role in the initial phase could be too toxic for long-term maintenance. It seldom makes sense to draw conclusions about the safety and efficacy of any given drug without considering in detail both the dosage and the schedule of administration.

At this time investigators must not pin their hopes on any single drug or approach but instead should strive to develop a variety of agents to attack HIV at different points. In bringing these drugs to a stage where they can benefit patients, there is a lesson to be drawn from the experience with AZT. Little more than two years elapsed from the time we first observed the drug's anti-HIV effect in our laboratory until the time AZT was approved as a prescription drug. We attribute this rapid development to the careful, scientifically controlled process by which the clinical trials were conducted. We cannot emphasize enough the importance of the controlled-trial method to the success of future therapies—and to much of what must be learned if AIDS is to be conquered.

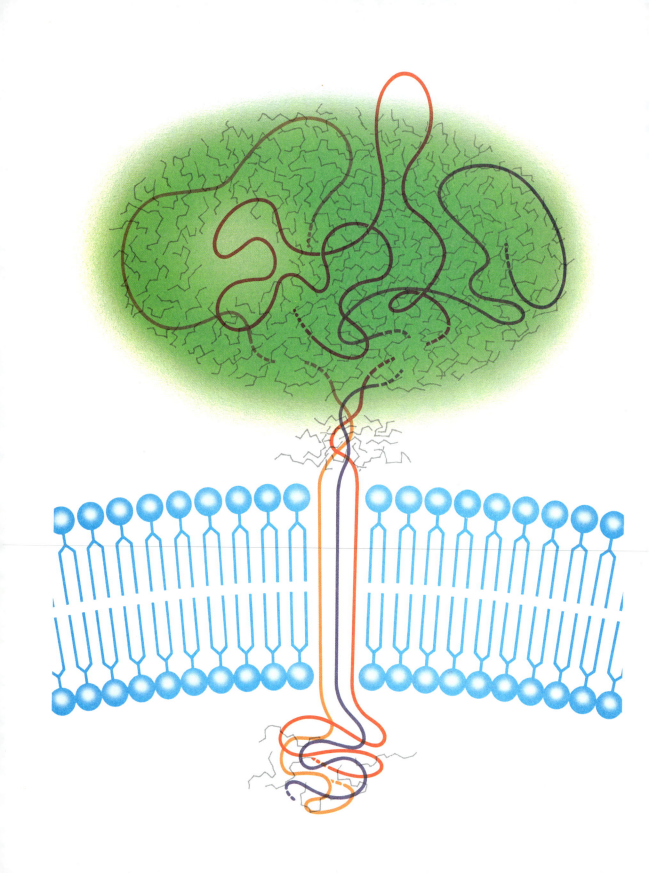

AIDS Vaccines

*Several candidates are being tested and more are on the way, but
success is far from assured. The life cycle of the virus and the
logistics of AIDS vaccine testing make HIV a foe without precedent.*

. . .

Thomas J. Matthews and Dani P. Bolognesi

The best way to combat any disease is to prevent it. Vaccination is the simplest, safest and most effective form of prevention, and vaccines have achieved legendary success against viruses. Because of vaccines the campaigns against smallpox and polio are resounding triumphs; the decline of yellow fever, measles, mumps and rubella is also due largely to vaccination. Against this backdrop of successes the human immunodeficiency virus (HIV) looms large. A vaccine against AIDS is perhaps the most formidable and urgent challenge facing virologists today.

Vaccine development has been a top priority of

AIDS research since HIV was conclusively shown to be the cause of the disease in 1984. Yet in spite of the millions of dollars and hundreds of scientists devoted to vaccine research, Surgeon General C. Everett Koop has warned the public not to expect a vaccine before the end of the century. Why not?

Researchers are daunted by three particulars: the devious nature of the virus itself, which can "hide" in cells, change the composition of its coat and install its own genes within the genes of its host; the lack of a good animal model for the disease, which slows investigations of vaccine strategies to combat these pioys, and the difficulties expected with clinical trials, which face scientific uncertainty, ethical concerns and possibly a shortage of volunteers.

Several vaccines are currently being tested in humans. It is much too early to pronounce on their performance, but most investigators are not optimistic. Yet no one is entertaining the idea of failure. A vaccine offers the best hope of stemming the AIDS crisis. A great deal has been learned about the virus since the first AIDS vaccines were designed, and we hope that tomorrow's vaccine candidates will have a better chance of defeating HIV if the current ones fail. Otherwise this decade in the shadow of AIDS will have been just a foretaste of the virus's ultimate

Figure 61 ENVELOPE PROTEIN is found on the surface of HIV and the cells it infects. The protein is thought to be a trimer of three virtually identical molecules, shown here in red, orange and purple. Much of the protein backbone is buried in a cloud of sugar molecules (*gray-green*). There is reason to believe a vaccine that mimics certain antigenic parts of the protein would induce a potent immune response. The immune system of people infected with HIV attacks the envelope protein, but the assault does not prevent disease. It may be that the sugar cloud protects vulnerable areas of the backbone, such as the pit (*left*) where the virus binds to its receptor, while less critical parts such as the loop (*right*) are exposed, perhaps as decoys.

impact on public health, behavior and economy across the globe.

A rich tradition of vaccine research guides the effort to develop an AIDS vaccine. Hundreds of years ago controlled inoculations of the pus from smallpox victims was used to immunize healthy individuals in the Far East and Middle East. Then in 1796 Edward Jenner found that cowpox virus could serve as a smallpox vaccine. His discovery led to the realization that the pathogenic organism itself need not be present to rally the immune system's defenses; only certain characteristic parts of an organism trigger an immune response. These parts (often proteins or protein fragments) are known as antigens.

Vaccines exploit the body's ability to "remember" an antigen. The first time the immune system encounters a given antigen in the course of infection it is caught unawares, but as a result of the encounter cells are generated that retain an immunological memory of the antigen for the lifetime of an individual. Consequently subsequent responses to the same invader are swifter and more potent. A vaccine introduces the antigen in a harmless form called an immunogen, so that the body becomes primed to fight off the infectious agent without risk of contracting the disease itself.

If the immune system is to defeat a pathogen, it must be able to attack the invader free in the blood as well as in association with cells. The immune response has two interrelated arms that combat infection on both fronts: a "humoral" response and a "cell-mediated" response. In the humoral response blood cells called B lymphocytes generate exquisitely specific antibody molecules that circulate in the blood and bind to antigens, thus nullifying the pathogen. The cell-mediated response involves "killer" T8 cells (also known as cytotoxic lymphocytes) that attack and destroy infected cells.

Central to both responses is another group of T cells, the T4 or "helper" cells. Helper cells send out chemical signals called lymphokines, which help to activate T- and B-cell populations and cause them to proliferate. The lymphokines from T4 cells also prompt the generation of antigen-specific "memory" cells for the T- and B-cell populations; it is these cells that are responsible for hastening and amplifying the immune response in subsequent encounters with the antigen (see Figure 62).

B cells and T cells interact with an antigen differently. B cells have receptors akin to antibodies that can recognize free antigen particles, but in order for a T cell to "see" an antigen the antigen must be presented on the surface of another cell. When a pathogen first invades the body, blood cells known as macrophages endocytose, or "swallow," the invader, process it and display its antigenic portions on their surface. T-cell receptors can bind to the processed antigens, and T cells thereby learn to identify infected cells, which bear the same processed antigens on their surface. Owing to these different modes of interaction, B cells usually recognize external antigens of a pathogen, whereas T cells can respond to both external antigens and internal components that become exposed during cellular processing. If a vaccine is to elicit humoral and cell-mediated immunity, it must contain immunogens that both arms of the immune system would see in the course of an ordinary infection.

V accine development is a greater challenge with HIV because the virus infects some of the same cells the vaccine needs to activate. While there is evidence that HIV can invade the central nervous system, the primary targets of infection are macrophages and T4 cells. Indeed, the macrophages, which can survive HIV infection, may serve as shuttles that carry HIV to T4 cells during the routine interactions of the two cell types. The T4 cells usually do not survive HIV infection. Because these cells play a critical role in the immune defense, on which any vaccine would rely, an AIDS vaccine would have to prevent the virus from becoming entrenched in T-cell and macrophage populations in the first place.

The vaccine would also have to halt the virus before it invades the central nervous system, where pathogens become invulnerable to immune attack. Furthermore, a vaccine must ensure that the immune system will recognize any and all of the innumerable HIV variants, and that protection will extend to all vaccine recipients regardless of age, gender and extent of exposure. And the vaccine must carry no risk of itself causing AIDS. Unless an immunogen has been shown to meet all these criteria, it cannot be called an AIDS vaccine per se; it is more correct to refer to it as a vaccine candidate.

In devising vaccine candidates, it is important to recognize that the way an immunogen is presented can have some bearing on its efficacy. Today vaccine researchers have a variety of options for presentation. Traditional vaccines are made of the virus itself, either killed or attenuated to render it harmless. These have been quite successful, presumably because whole virus is a potent immunogen. Vaccines against measles, mumps and rubella all contain live, attenuated virus, whereas rabies vaccines are made from killed virus. There are both attenuated- and killed-virus polio vaccines.

Exposing people to whole virus is not entirely without risk: in the U.S., for example, a handful of children every year get polio from attenuated polio vaccines. In most cases vaccines using antigenic subunits rather than the pathogen itself would be preferable because they eliminate the threat of inadvertent infection. The technology for producing such vaccines has evolved only recently, and a subunit vaccine against hepatitis B, made by Merck Sharp & Dohme, has already been approved in the U.S.

Subunit vaccines have several drawbacks of their own. Subunits by themselves can be invisible to the immune system and must often be combined with some kind of vehicle to improve their immunogenicity. For example, the subunit may be complexed with a so-called adjuvant, which attracts the immune system's attention by causing inflammation or by acting as an antigen in its own right. In addition the subunit used in a vaccine must be carefully chosen, because not all components of a pathogen represent beneficial immunological targets. Some may even induce inappropriate responses that preempt protective ones.

In the case of AIDS there is no precedent lending support to any one of these approaches. Hence workers are pursuing a number of strategies in designing their AIDS vaccines.

Indeed, lack of a precedent plagues quite a few aspects of AIDS vaccine research. HIV belongs to a class of viruses, called retroviruses, with which the research community has had limited experience. Human retroviruses were discovered less than a decade ago and animal retroviruses have never been deemed significant enough to provide a practical incentive for vaccine development. The only real field trials of a retroviral vaccine were done in cats, with a vaccine against feline leukemia. In these trials a subunit vaccine provided partial protection; experimental vaccines using attenuated virus or better-defined subunits with improved adjuvants have shown greater promise. But now that the search for an AIDS vaccine has taken center stage, it has become painfully clear how difficult the development of vaccines against retroviruses can be.

Retroviruses, like a few other types of virus, can insert their own genes into the genes of the cells they infect, thereby establishing a permanent infection. Even if a cell is not actively producing virus particles, it may still harbor "dormant" retroviral genes. Such a cell might remain invisible to the immune system because no viral antigens would be displayed on its surface. Hence eradicating a retroviral infection could prove to be impossible, although a vaccine might still be able to stimulate the immune system enough to keep the virus from causing disease. For example, in studies of mouse leukemia, a retroviral disease, Werner Schäfer and his colleagues at the Max Planck Institute for Virus Research in Tübingen found that an experimental vaccine could protect the animals from disease, but the virus reappeared late in life, when the animals' immune systems began to falter.

The virus did not cause leukemia when it reemerged, and so it seems that a total blockade of infection may not be necessary for long-term protection against a retroviral disease. Indeed, most successful vaccines protect against disease rather than infection. There is one way, however, in which a retroviral infection differs from most other viral infections for which vaccines exist: retroviral genes contain regulatory elements that can disrupt a cell's normal growth patterns. In other words, the genes can cause cancer.

Thus the mere presence of retroviral genes in the body is a real cause for concern. This raises the daunting possibility that an AIDS vaccine may have to achieve a complete blockade of infection. It is not practical to expect such a blockade from any vaccine, and so vaccine developers hope that some degree of infection can be tolerated. In any case, the option of an attenuated whole-virus vaccine has been all but eliminated, since disabled retroviral genetic material could induce malignancy even if it could not orchestrate the production of virus particles.

Unfortunately the problems surrounding vaccination against HIV are not limited to those associated with its being a retrovirus. HIV has several features of its own that make it a singular opponent.

Perhaps the most infamous characteristic of the virus is its propensity to mutate. This tendency is particularly pronounced in the gene that codes for its envelope protein, gp120. Vaccine developers have focused a great deal of attention on gp120

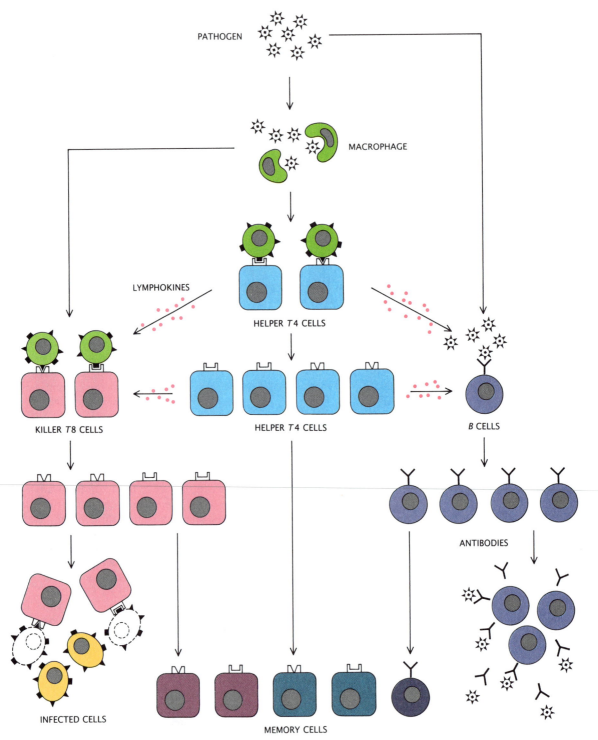

PATHOGEN

MACROPHAGE

LYMPHOKINES

HELPER T4 CELLS

KILLER T8 CELLS

HELPER T4 CELLS

B CELLS

ANTIBODIES

INFECTED CELLS

MEMORY CELLS

because it is displayed on the surface of both the virus and infected cells, which makes it a likely target for an immune response. The virus probably confounds the immune system by continually varying the sequence of amino acids that make up this outermost protein. If a vaccine is to exploit the immunogenicity of the gp120 molecule, more will have to be learned about the diversity of gp120 variants.

Another troublesome aspect of HIV infection has been brought to light by recent evidence that virus particles can be trapped in vesicles — enclosed pockets in the cell cytoplasm — without betraying their presence through viral proteins on the cell surface. Without surface antigens the cell-mediated arm of the immune system cannot detect the infection and will not attack the cell. Ashley T. Haase of the University of Minnesota Medical School applied the term "Trojan horse" to describe such evasive behavior in animal retroviruses; if a virus adopts this strategy, the immune system never gets a glimpse of it. Thus the virus might be passed between cells in an individual or even transmitted from one person to another while remaining hidden.

In addition the virus has a remarkable affinity for the cell-surface protein, known as CD4, to which it binds (see Chapter 7, "HIV Infection: The Cellular Picture," by Jonathan N. Weber and Robin A. Weiss). Antibodies induced by a vaccine will have to overcome this powerful affinity if they are to impede binding. Antibodies to the part of the virus that binds to the CD4 receptor could mechanically obstruct the binding process, but that approach has its own hazards. In particular, antibodies to the virus's combining site actually resemble the CD4 receptor, and if, as often happens, a second round of antibodies is produced against the first, they

would in turn mimic the binding site on the virus. Consequently the second round of antibodies could attack CD4, incapacitating or destroying the very cells that are already under siege from the virus.

Recent evidence that people infected with HIV make antibodies to CD4 lends credibility to this scenario. Such a phenomenon, which is known as an autoimmune reaction, could occur with any vaccine, but in existing vaccines the combining site of the virus need not be the primary antigenic constituent. Furthermore, there is reason to believe that vaccines representing other sites on the HIV envelope protein might also trigger an autoimmune response, because some parts of the envelope are known to mimic normal cell-surface markers.

The fact that HIV attacks the cells that are responsible for defeating infection adds its own twist to vaccine development. In particular, some investigators are concerned that a vaccine could actually enhance the infectivity of the virus. Certain cells of the immune system have receptors that bind to antibodies opposite the antigen-binding region. Macrophages are among these cells, and macrophages are a target of HIV infection. Antibodies attached to free virus could therefore be attracted to macrophages, increasing the chances that a macrophage will become infected. Hence raising antibodies to HIV by means of a vaccine could conceivably facilitate rather than deter the spread of the virus. It is still not clear that this effect actually potentiates infection during natural exposure to the virus.

Does such a recalcitrant virus have an Achilles' heel? Even though examples of successful vaccines against retroviruses are lacking, vaccine developers have challenged other formidable viruses and won. The virus that causes hepatitis B, for instance, also has sophisticated strategies for escaping immune destruction and can establish persistent latent and chronic infections. Likewise, HIV is probably not invulnerable.

Components of the immune system have proved able to neutralize the virus in the test tube, and people who are infected with HIV initially launch strong humoral and cellular assaults. They make antibodies against components of the viral envelope, and their killer T cells recognize internal components of the virus as well as parts of the envelope. These defenses may hold the virus in check for several years (see Chapter 6, "HIV Infection: The Clinical Picture," by Robert R. Redfield and Donald S. Burke). Yet these people eventually develop AIDS

Figure 62 IMMUNE ATTACK on a pathogen involves both humoral (B cell) and the cell-mediated (T cell) responses. Macrophages engulf the invader and display its internal (*square*) and external (*triangular*) antigenic components to receptors on T cells. The "helper" T4 cells multiply and produce lymphokines (*red*). Interaction with macrophages and T4 cells causes "killer" T8 cells to mature and roam the bloodstream, destroying infected cells. Meanwhile external antigens on the pathogen interact with receptors on B cells. If the B cells receive lymphokine signals, they proliferate and secrete antibodies that bind to the antigens and neutralize them. Antigen-specific "memory" cells are also generated; these enable the immune system to combat the same invader more effectively in future encounters.

anyway. The immune system fights back; it just does not fight hard enough.

The trick is to discover which part of HIV elicits the most powerful natural immune response and amplify that response enough to overcome the virus. It might even be possible to teach the immune system to recognize antigenic sites that are ordinarily hidden by the virus. At present there is no reason to narrow the scope of investigation to any particular piece of the virus, but most studies focus on the gp120 envelope protein.

The *gp* stands for "glycoprotein"; in its natural state the protein is wrapped on itself like string and covered with a cloud of sugar (glyco-) molecules. It is anchored to the surface of the virus or an infected cell by a protein called gp41, which penetrates the surface membrane. The glycoproteins are derived from a precursor called gp160.

Most of gp120 is obscured from immunological sight by the cloud of sugar; the sugar molecules are poorly antigenic at best, because they are made by the host cell. The topography of the molecule, as far as it is known, is distinguished by two features: a pit or cleft where the protein binds to CD4, and a loop that protrudes from the sugar cloud. What is known about these two features has largely been inferred from observations of their immunogenic properties. For example, it is difficult to raise antibodies against the CD4 binding site in the laboratory, and so it has been assumed that the site is recessed within the molecule and probably shrouded with sugar. The loop, on the other hand, is highly immunogenic and is therefore thought to be exposed.

Antibodies against both regions have been successful in blocking early steps in viral infection. A common sequence of events characterizes the initial encounter. First gp120 binds to the CD4 receptor on an uninfected cell; then gp41 becomes anchored in the adjoining membrane; next the two membranes begin to fuse, and the virus spills its contents into the cell. An immune reaction that interferes with any of these steps—binding, anchorage or fusion—could prevent infection.

In some ways the CD4 binding site of gp120 would seem to be the ideal immunogen. Although, as mentioned above, it could provoke an autoimmune response, it is integral to the virus's function and is highly conserved; that is, it does not vary much from strain to strain. The process by which the immune system gets at the CD4 site is probably complex, requiring prolonged exposure to the virus, since people who are infected with HIV do not start

making antibodies that interfere with CD4 binding until about a year after they become infected. A vaccine making the CD4 site conspicuous might expedite the immune reaction. There is a problem, however, in that the antibodies that block binding do not block infection as well as one would expect.

On the other hand, antibodies that interfere with postbinding steps are very good at blocking infection. Scott D. Putney, James R. Rusche and Kashi Javaherian at the Repligen Corporation, Flossie Wong-Staal and Robert C. Gallo at the National Cancer Institute and our group at the Duke University Medical Center with our colleagues Thomas J. Palker and Barton F. Haynes have demonstrated that such antibodies bind to the loop portion of the envelope protein. Indeed, the loop seems to be easily and rapidly recognized by the immune system and is therefore called the immunodominant site on gp120. People infected with HIV produce antibodies against the loop in the earlier stages of the infection; these antibodies might be responsible for controlling the spread of the virus during the disease's latent period.

Interestingly, the loop is also one of the most variable regions of the protein, and no one has been able to ascertain its function. Might the loop be a decoy? Its prominence could divert the immune system's attention from less accessible and more essential sites, while its hypervariability would enable it to dodge the immune response it draws (a single change in the loop's amino acid sequence creates a different antibody specificity). It might be possible to overcome the variability with a vaccine that would anticipate all mutated forms—the equivalent of a "universal loop."

Even as investigators puzzle out strategies for new vaccine candidates, the first crop of AIDS vaccines is being tested in human subjects. So far too little has been learned from the clinical trials to guide current research or hint at the superiority of one approach over the other. Most workers, however, are employing the subunit approach, and most are using whole envelope proteins as the subunit.

At least two modes of presentation are being considered to ensure that the immune system does not overlook the envelope antigen. The subunit can be complexed with an adjuvant, or the gene for the subunit can be inserted into an attenuated virus that will express the HIV protein in its own envelope. The first AIDS vaccine candidate to enter clinical trials in the U.S. is a gp160 subunit combined with

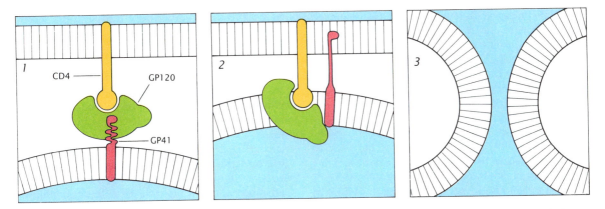

Figure 63 STEPS IN HIV INFECTION include binding, anchorage and fusion, which are mediated by envelope components of the virus. Initially the virus associates with a receptor called CD4 on an uninfected cell. The pit of gp120 binds to CD4 (1); then gp41 becomes anchored in the cell membrane (2), holding the membranes in proximity so that they can fuse (3). Infected cells fuse with uninfected cells in much the same way. The loop probably has a role in the process, but it has not been identified.

the simple household chemical alum as an adjuvant. The vaccine, which is made by MicroGeneSys, Inc., in West Haven, Conn., entered trials in October, 1987, at the National Institute of Allergy and Infectious Diseases (NIAID). Results gathered so far are ambiguous, but investigators think increasing dose levels may improve the candidate vaccine's performance. In Switzerland a gp120-adjuvant vaccine made by the Chiron Corporation of Emeryville, Calif., and the Swiss pharmaceutical company Ciba-Geigy AG has been approved for human trials. The trials will include about two dozen volunteers.

For subunit-adjuvant vaccines the type of adjuvant employed is often critical to the vaccine's performance. Immune recognition might well be improved by complexing the subunit with more sophisticated adjuvants, such as artificial membranes called liposomes or so-called immune-stimulating complexes. Work by Bror Morein of the University of Uppsala has demonstrated the efficacy of this approach with other immunogens, and its extension to experimental AIDS vaccines has already shown promise.

The most impressive results to date, however, have been obtained from trials of a subunit vaccine

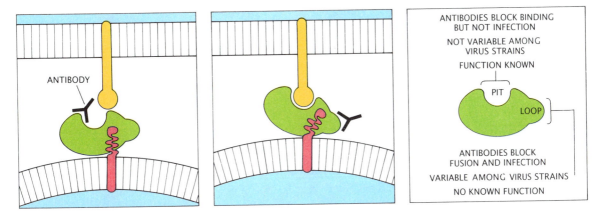

Figure 64 ANTIBODIES BLOCK STEPS IN INFECTION if they bind to the pit or the loop of the gp120 protein. Antibodies against the pit block binding (box at left), and antibodies against the loop block fusion (middle box). The two sites have distinctly different characteristics that affect their suitability as immunogens, or substances that provoke an immune response (box at right).

candidate using an attenuated vaccinia (cowpox) virus vector. These trials were conducted in Zaire, where the virus is endemic. They were the first test of an AIDS vaccine in humans; it took many by surprise when the head of the research group, Daniel Zagury of the University of Paris, announced that he had inoculated himself along with the first volunteers in November, 1986.

Zagury and his colleagues utilize a vaccinia technology pioneered by Bernard Moss of the NIAID to create the vector for the initial inoculation. They follow the inoculation with boosters consisting of purified gp160 and a special preparation of T cells: cells that were taken previously from the same individual, infected with the HIV-vaccinia vector and then killed before reinjection.

This protocol produces potent humoral and cellular anti-HIV activity of long duration. It is too complicated to be feasible as a vaccine strategy, but it demonstrates that immunity to HIV can be achieved in human beings. Zagury is looking for a simpler way to elicit the same response. Meanwhile results are just beginning to come in from U.S. trials of another gp160-vaccinia vaccine made by Oncogen, a Seattle, Wash., subsidiary of the Bristol-Myers Co.

Allan L. Goldstein and his colleagues at the George Washington University School of Medicine and Health Sciences were among the first investigators to design a subunit vaccine based on an internal component of the virus rather than an envelope antigen. Their vaccine candidate, called HGP-30, is made by Viral Technologies, Inc., in Washington, D.C. It is undergoing clinical trials in London and awaiting approval for trials in the U.S. HGP-30 mimics a part of the protein p17, which lines the inside of HIV's envelope. The protein is probably exposed to immune attack during processing by macrophages and infected cells: people who are infected with HIV produce antibodies against p17, and their infected cells often display the protein on their surface.

A somewhat more esoteric approach is under investigation in England by Angus G. Dalgleish of the Clinical Research Centre in Harrow and Ronald C. Kennedy of the Southwest Foundation for Biomedical Research in San Antonio, Tex. The two are part of an international consortium including the Imperial Cancer Research Fund, University College London and the Becton Dickinson Monoclonal Center, Inc. Their approach assumes that antibodies that mimic the receptor for the pathogen—in this case CD4—will compete very well with the receptor in binding the pathogen. Such antibodies can be generated with an immunogen that represents the "internal image" of the receptor the way a key represents the internal image of a lock. Hence inoculations of antibodies against CD4 should raise a population of antibodies, known as anti-idiotype antibodies, that resemble CD4. These could tie up free virus in the blood. Indeed, CD4 made by genetic engineering is known to inhibit HIV infection in vitro, and the substance itself has been slated for clinical trials. In London two individuals have already received anti-idiotype inoculations; preliminary results have not been reported.

An experimental vaccine made from killed HIV has been prepared by Jonas Salk and his colleagues at the Salk Institute for Biological Studies. Because of the risks of inoculation with whole HIV, the vaccine would be appropriate only for boosting the immune reaction of people who are already infected with the virus. Such so-called postexposure vaccines have been somewhat effective in rabies-virus infections, but their efficacy has not been demonstrated for retroviral infections. Salk has administered his vaccine to roughly a dozen individuals with early symptoms of AIDS. So far he reports no pronounced benefits.

Although encouraging results are in short supply, it is remarkable in itself that so many candidate HIV vaccines have reached the human testing phase just four years after the cause of AIDS was discovered. This progress attests to the arduous efforts of vaccine researchers here and in other countries, faced with one of the most intractable viral diseases in medical history. Yet AIDS vaccine researchers are still working in the dark compared with their predecessors in at least one respect: they have no good animal model for the disease.

Other human viral diseases have analogues in laboratory animals, but most animals do not get AIDS from HIV. No one knows why. Considerable effort is being spent to find out, because the answer would probably reveal how human beings could defend themselves against the virus. Chimpanzees can be infected with the virus, but chimps infected years ago still show no signs of illness.

Several advances announced earlier this year offer hope of an alternative. Macaque monkeys infected with HIV-2—a variant of HIV found predominantly in West Africa—contracted AIDS and thus became the first subhuman animal ever to get a

TYPE OF VACCINE	RESEARCH GROUP	TYPE OF IMMUNOGEN	IMMUNOGENS TESTED IN PEOPLE
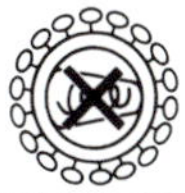 KILLED VIRUS	Salk Institute for Biological Studies University of California at Davis	Whole or disrupted inactivated HIV with genetic material removed	Whole inactivated HIV in infected people
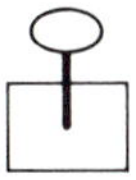 HIV SUBUNIT WITH ADJUVANT	Genentech Inc. MicroGeneSys, Inc. Immuno AG National Cancer Institute Repligen Corporation/Merck Sharp & Dohme Duke University Medical Center Ciba-Geigy AG/Chiron Corporation Smith Kline & French Laboratories Merieux Institute/ Cambridge Bioscience Corporation Viral Technologies, Inc. University of Uppsala Wistar Institute of Anatomy and Biology University of Paris Southwest Foundation for Biomedical Research	HIV envelope, pieces of envelope proteins or other structural antigens made by genetically engineered cells or synthesized in the laboratory	gp160, gp120 and synthetic fragment of p17
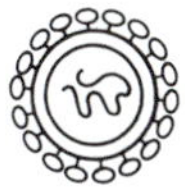 HIV SUBUNIT IN VIRUS VECTOR	University of Paris Bristol-Myers, Co. Merieux Institute/Transgene S. A. Wyeth Laboratories National Institute of Allergy and Infectious Diseases National Cancer Institute	Gene for HIV envelope protein inserted in vaccinia virus or adenovirus, or cells infected with HIV/ vaccinia recombinant	Vaccinia/HIV recombinant and cells infected with recombinant
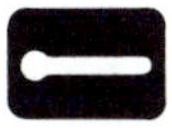 ANTI-IDIOTYPE	Clinical Research Center/Southwest Foundation for Biomedical Research/ Becton Dickinson Monoclonal Center, Inc./ Imperial Cancer Research Fund/ University College London	Antibody against CD4	Antibody against CD4

Figure 65 VACCINE RESEARCH encompasses several different strategies, in various phases of testing. Subunit vaccines are by far the most popular; they are made by combining a piece of HIV with an adjuvant or by inserting a gene for an HIV protein among the genes of a harmless virus "vector." Anti-idiotype vaccines consist of antibodies carrying an internal image of the CD4 receptor, meant to evoke another set of antibodies that look like CD4 and compete with it for binding to HIV. Killed HIV vaccines, which immunize with whole or disrupted virus, have been deemed too risky for inoculating people who have not already been exposed to HIV. This partial list is by no means exhaustive. Many of the groups are exploring more than one approach and collaborating with one another and groups that are not listed.

disease from a human retrovirus. The finding has excited the research community because it demonstrates that animals can get AIDS, and macaques are much easier to work with than chimps. It is not clear, however, to what extent the lessons learned from HIV-2 can be applied to its commoner and possibly more pathogenic relative, HIV-1. There is also evidence that rabbits infected with HIV display some signs of disease.

Other retroviruses may serve as HIV analogues. Simian immunodeficiency virus (SIV), for example, causes a disease much like AIDS in monkeys. Unfortunately the first test of an SIV vaccine, at the New England Regional Primate Center in Southboro, Mass., failed. Retroviruses that cause immunodeficiency syndromes in cows and cats are also being investigated.

In the meantime there is no way to establish criteria for the efficacy of AIDS vaccines before injecting them in humans. When other vaccines were about to enter clinical trials, investigators had a good idea of what kind of immune response was necessary to fend off the disease. But no one knows what constitutes protective immunity against AIDS. Is it a certain titer of antibodies, a particular level of killer-T-cell activity, or some synergistic interaction between the two?

And when can a given immunization be judged a success? Ethical obligations require that clinicians counsel their volunteers to avoid behavior that could lead to HIV infection, and so a low incidence of AIDS in these people could reflect "safe sex" practices rather than the action of an experimental vaccine. How can anyone be sure a vaccine has warded off disease short of injecting the vaccine recipient with HIV and observing the consequences? Given that the disease's latency period can last for five years, how long should doctors wait before concluding that protection has been achieved?

Clinicians also expect to be confronted with a shortage of trial volunteers, first because healthy people may be understandably reluctant to try a vaccine that has no demonstrated efficacy, and second because there simply may not be enough people in high-risk categories to provide statistically significant results. (People in low-risk groups have such a slim chance of encountering the virus that it would be virtually impossible to demonstrate efficacy in a reasonable period of time.)

The recruitment problem will get worse, not better, as more vaccines are developed. Each vaccine candidate requires from 50 to 100 high-risk volunteers for the first phase of trials, and the final phase of testing could involve thousands of people. Each volunteer can take part in only one trial. Massive testing is theoretically feasible in areas of the Third World where the virus is endemic, but such a program would be complicated by political, social and logistical considerations. Should a limit be placed on the number of vaccines that can win approval for human testing?

Finally, the liability issues surrounding the testing of an AIDS vaccine remain unresolved. Leaders of corporate research, such as Maurice R. Hilleman of the Merck Institute for Therapeutic Research, have warned that the uncertainty surrounding the risks of vaccine-related injuries and compensation for them could ultimately hinder development. Some framework must be drawn up that will allow companies to proceed with vaccine development and testing without courting litigious disaster.

In surveying all the difficulties bearing on the development of an AIDS vaccine, it would be easy enough to lose heart. But at one time the situation must have appeared just as hopeless to Jenner. A vaccine against HIV is the highest aspiration of AIDS research and would represent a triumph for virology as well.

Small wonder that scientists from all over the world have become engaged in this effort. Many of them participate in Gallo's international HIVAC (HIV vaccine) group, which brings together workers from 10 different countries. Major vaccine research programs have also been established in Great Britain, France, Sweden, Germany and Japan. In the U.S. the Public Health Service has drawn up a plan for vaccine development and evaluation that includes National Cooperative Vaccine Development Groups, which will coordinate collaboration between government, industry and academic efforts. Many other investigators are independently pooling their expertise in a multitude of virus types, in the mechanisms of gene regulation and in the workings of the immune system. We believe HIV cannot outwit such a combination.

The Social Dimensions of AIDS

AIDS exposes the hidden weaknesses in human society; how the epidemic is dealt with will have a profound effect on society's future. A crucial issue is protection from discrimination.

. . .

Harvey V. Fineberg

The AIDS epidemic exposes hidden vulnerabilities in the human condition that are both biological and social. AIDS prompts courageous and generous acts, and it provokes mean-spirited and irrational responses. AIDS throws new light on traditional questions of value, compels a fresh look at the performance of the institutions we depend on and brings society to a crossroads for collective action that may, with the passage of years, mark a key measure of our time.

In the seven years since AIDS was recognized, the epidemic has touched on almost all aspects of society. Its reach extends to every social institution, from families, schools and communities to businesses, courts of law, the military and Federal, state and local governments. It has also had a profound impact on the way science, medicine and public health are practiced in the world.

Through its association with sex, blood, drugs and death, AIDS evokes basic human fears and inhibitions. In her book *Illness as Metaphor* Susan Sontag writes: "Although the way in which disease mystifies is set against a backdrop of new expectations, the disease itself . . . arouses thoroughly old-fashioned kinds of dread. Any disease that is treated as a mystery and acutely enough feared will

be felt morally, if not literally, contagious. . . . Contact with someone afflicted with a disease regarded as a mysterious malevolency inevitably feels like a trespass; worse, like the violation of a taboo."

Although she was reflecting on cancer, Sontag's words are even more appropriate for AIDS, a condition that is literally as well as morally contagious. The contagion is compounded by the stigma attached to the behaviors most prominently associated with HIV infection in the U.S.: homosexual intercourse and intravenous drug use. Knowledge of HIV and its mode of spread, convincing as it is to scientists and epidemiologists, is not powerful enough to fully dissolve the public sense of mystery and old-fashioned dread. The protective garb needlessly donned by workers transporting a person with AIDS is reminiscent of the costume worn by physicians treating plague victims in 18th-century France. People known to be infected with HIV have lost jobs, homes and friends. Children with AIDS have been denied access to public schools and in 1987 a major air carrier temporarily refused to transport patients with AIDS. People with AIDS have even been denied transportation to the grave, as some funeral directors have refused to handle their corpses.

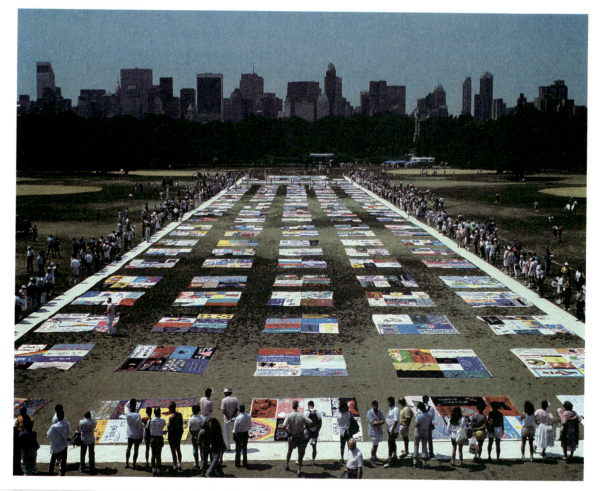

Figure 66 NEW YORK MEMORIAL QUILT is a reminder of lives lost to AIDS. Each panel represents a resident of the New York area who died of the disease. The quilt, shown here in Central Park, will be incorporated in the national Names Project AIDS quilt.

AIDS is a modern affliction. The AIDS epidemic was fomented by changes in social mores and lifestyle that are unique to the latter part of the 20th century: urbanization in Africa, gay consciousness and liberation in the U.S., development of technologies for the preservation and shipment of blood-clotting factors for hemophiliacs, and modern air travel. Unlike some other infectious diseases, the AIDS virus is carried and transmitted by the human host; there is no apparent insect or other animal vector and the virus has no special climatic requirements. Because AIDS spreads directly from one person to another, the disease is—at least potentially—a universal problem. It is the one contemporary disease that is keenly felt as an urgent problem in both industrialized and less developed countries.

HIV is insidious. It corrupts vital body fluids, turning blood and semen from sources of life into instruments of death. The virus insinuates itself into the genetic material of selected cells, where it may remain quiescent for prolonged periods of time. When it is active, the virus gradually undermines the body's immune system, eventually rendering it vulnerable to opportunistic infections. During the latency period, which may average eight years or longer, the patient feels perfectly well yet is capable of transmitting the virus to others. HIV infection remains at the present time incurable, a pointed

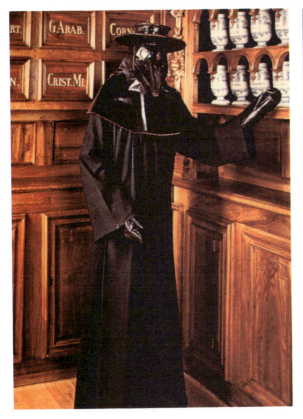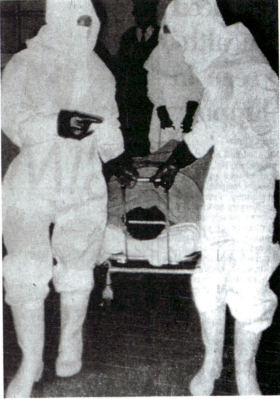

Figure 67 FEAR OF CONTAGION was a legitimate concern during the plague outbreak of 1720, when French physicians wore special garments to avoid infection from respiratory droplets and fleas (*left*). Such fear is unjustified in the case of AIDS, but it remains widespread. Two ambulance workers in Hong Kong (*right*) donned protective suits to transport an AIDS patient.

reminder of humanity's thrall to the tyranny of nature.

Because of its association with sex and its long latency period, AIDS has altered our thinking and prompted much discussion about human relations, love and sexuality. The AIDS epidemic has heightened awareness of homosexuality in our society, promoting understanding and tolerance in some and reinforcing aversion in others. The ease and readiness with which many now speak in public about homosexuality, sexual practices, the use of condoms and similar matters could hardly have been foreseen 10 years ago. The willingness of so many to see formerly taboo subjects presented in the media testifies to the extent to which AIDS has affected the standards of public discourse. The National AIDS Awareness Test presented on U.S. television in September, 1987, was introduced with the warning that some viewers might be offended; viewers were assured that nearly all those surveyed during the program's preparation believed the subject should be aired. Soon such reassurances about the need to discuss AIDS candidly will seem superfluous, because it will be obvious that we can no longer afford to live according to old inhibitions in discussing sexual practices and other risk factors that relate to this disease.

The HIV epidemic is marked by sharp variation in geographic, racial and gender composition. Globally three disparate patterns in the distribution of AIDS have been discerned. In the U.S. and other industrialized countries with large numbers of cases, the predominant modes of spread have been through homosexual activities and intravenous drug use, and the ratio of male to female cases is approximately 10 to one. In central, eastern and southern Africa and in parts of the Caribbean, heterosexual spread predominates, with a male to female ratio of about one to one. In these economically disadvantaged parts of the world perinatal transmission is high and blood-borne spread continues to be a significant problem because of inadequate or absent screening procedures. In some parts of the world, such as eastern Europe, the Middle East and Asia, very few cases have been reported. Officials in these countries tend to ascribe most of their cases to travel, or to contacts with travelers from endemic areas, much as cases of heterosexual transmission in the U.S. are mainly attributed to contact with individuals who are bisexual or intravenous drug users. In neither setting should the current pattern offer much reassurance about the future.

Within the U.S. the geographic distribution of AIDS is highly uneven, minorities are disproportionately represented and intravenous drug use plays an increasing role in transmission. By mid-1988 the U.S. had counted 65,000 cases. More than half the states have reported fewer than 400 cases each, with a range of from fewer than 10 in each of the Dakotas to more than 16,000 in New York. The distribution is expected to be lopsided for some time, but the rest of the country is tending to catch up with the epicenters of the epidemic in New York City and San Francisco. In 1984 these cities had half of all the AIDS cases in the U.S.; in 1987 they had only 25 percent of new cases.

In San Francisco 85 percent of all reported cases of AIDS are among homosexual men who deny use of intravenous drugs; in contrast, 36 percent of cases in New York City are related to intravenous drug use. The majority of infected women in the U.S., who constituted more than 10 percent of the new cases of AIDS in the first half of 1988, are exposed by intravenous drug use, and an estimated 70 percent of HIV infection in newborns is related to intravenous drugs. The epidemic has hit minority communities particularly hard. Blacks and Hispanics constitute about 20 percent of the U.S. population yet make up 40 percent of AIDS cases.

The principal means by which the spread of HIV infection can be stemmed—education and altered behavior patterns—are at once clear and elusive. Behavior related to sex and drugs is biologically based, socially conditioned and resistant to change. In some of the homosexual communities most severely affected by AIDS, particularly those in San Francisco, sustained and intensive educational efforts have been rewarded by striking changes in behavior and arrested transmission of the HIV.

Yet the gap between knowledge and personal action remains wide. In a national poll conducted in August, 1987, more than 90 percent of Americans knew they could contract AIDS from having sex or sharing needles with an infected person. Yet when they were asked about the possibility of contracting AIDS themselves, 90 percent of all respondents said they viewed their own risk as low or nonexistent. Surveys taken after a 1987 New York City advertising campaign for AIDS prevention showed that 80 percent of the respondents agreed that sexually active people should carry condoms and women should tell their sexual partner to use a condom. Yet the reported numbers and frequency of sexual contacts in the preceding month had not changed and more than 60 percent of those surveyed said they had failed to use a condom more than just some of the time. If the effectiveness of education is to be measured by behavioral change, success will not come easily.

Health officials are particularly concerned about the increase in HIV infection among intravenous drug users. In 1987 they represented 16 percent of new AIDS cases; in the first half of 1988 that number had grown to 21 percent. Serum surveys reveal that 50 percent or more of the intravenous drug users in New York City have antibodies to HIV. Of the more than 1.2 million intravenous drug users in the U.S., fewer than 250,000 are estimated to be in treatment at any one time. In some cities the waiting period for those who seek treatment is longer than six months.

Such bleak statistics led the President's Commission on the Human Immunodeficiency Virus Epidemic to call for 2,500 new treatment sites and an additional annual investment of $1.5 billion in drug-control programs. At the community level, street workers in a number of cities are attempting to protect drug users from HIV by showing them how to clean their needles and syringes with dilute bleach solution. Following the lead of European cities, Portland, Ore., recently undertook a trial program of providing drug users with sterile needles in exchange for dirty ones. Similar proposals have been made in Boston and New York, where they have met with considerable controversy. Critics oppose any appearance of state-sanctioned drug use and doubt the efficacy of exchange programs; advocates hold the preservation of life as a higher value and argue in favor of trial programs.

Another controversial proposal to stem the spread of AIDS, considered by legislatures in more than 30 states, is mandatory premarital screening for antibodies to HIV. Public-health officials and others have argued strenuously against such measures, saying that universal premarital screening would be counterproductive at this time. They point out that such tests would yield few truly positive results in a low-risk population, yet would overwhelm test sites, produce needless anxiety among those tested and waste resources. For the most part the arguments against screening have been convincing, although several states, including Illinois, adopted such legislation last year. Early experience in Illinois, however, bears out the predictions of public-health officials, suggesting that there are many problems and few benefits associated with universal premarital screening.

As with many other public-health measures, decisions about HIV screening tests should be reexamined in light of the changing dynamics of the AIDS epidemic. As the prevalence of the disease increases, the ratio of false-positive results to true positives will decrease. (The reasons for the decrease are technical and somewhat beyond the scope of this article, but basically they stem from the increase of the fraction of the population that is infected.) Technical advances in testing and improvements in the quality assurance of laboratories where the tests are conducted will also enhance performance. If there are advances in therapy, such as development of an effective and safe treatment for the asymptomatic HIV carrier, then increased emphasis on screening would be more desirable.

Containing the spread of HIV infection in the U.S. today requires special attention to minority communities. Some black leaders have been understandably reluctant to add the stigma of AIDS to the burden of racism. An increasing number of them, however, are now prepared to take up the challenge of stopping the spread of HIV. The singer Dionne Warwick, for example, who was appointed Ambassador of Health by the U.S. Department of Health and Human Services in 1987, has made AIDS one of her highest priorities. She has focused her efforts on the minority community, enlisting the support of other celebrities to raise money for education, research and patient services. In fiscal 1988 the U.S. Centers for Disease Control spent $10 million on state programs to combat HIV in minority commu-

nities, with $3 million earmarked for community organizations. Some private foundations are also giving special attention to community-based programs. With the support of the Kaiser Family Foundation in Menlo Park, Calif., the School of Medicine at Morehouse College in Atlanta is managing a health-promotion program that includes AIDS education for minority communities in 15 eastern states.

Intravenous drug use flourishes in areas that are burdened by unemployment, homelessness, welfare dependency, prostitution, crime, school dropout and teen-age pregnancy. These conditions are so intertwined that no one of them can be solved in the long term without providing the fundamental infrastructure—jobs, schools and housing—needed by any community. Such an infrastructure would go a long way toward creating the individual self-respect, dignity and hope for the future that can forestall the turning to drugs in the first place.

Perhaps the specter of AIDS will arouse the nation's determination to face up to those realities. The darker possibility is that racial discrimination will become camouflaged under the delusion that AIDS is a problem for poor blacks and Hispanics and need not concern white, middle-class America. It is as dangerous and shortsighted for whites to view AIDS as a minority disease as it has been for blacks and Hispanics to view AIDS as a white homosexual disease. Anyone who engages in risky activities, including heterosexual sex outside of a monogamous relationship, stands a chance of becoming infected. The risk in some geographic areas and some population groups is now exceedingly low, but no one can foresee with confidence the course of the HIV epidemic over the next 25 years.

The advent of AIDS has indelibly marked the practice of medicine in the U.S. The adoption of universal precautions by many hospitals means that the blood and certain body fluids of all patients are to be regarded as potentially infectious to health-care workers. Some hospitals in cities with large numbers of AIDS patients have established dedicated clinical units to care for hospitalized AIDS patients. At the other extreme, a private pediatric hospital recently announced that it was not going to admit HIV-infected children. If an admitted child is found to harbor the AIDS virus, then the child will be transferred to another hospital. The same hospital also began a systematic testing program for its employees to ensure that the entire institution would remain free of HIV infection. Many hospitals frankly do not want AIDS to drive away their "real" patients: those who can most easily pay.

The stress of AIDS on health-care workers can be tremendous. Doctors and nurses face young and desperately ill patients suffering from a disease for which there is at present no cure. The medical and insurance systems around them resist the kind of counseling, home treatment and hospice care that the patient may need most. The doctor may be caught in conflicts between patients, lovers, family and friends; other AIDS patients may have no evident social support at all.

What is more, health-care workers have legitimate concerns about occupational exposure to HIV, although that risk is low. (Available data suggest that the risk of transmission from a single needle stick is less than half of 1 percent.) Some may harbor prejudice or moral judgments about the behavior of their patients. Fewer physicians today are choosing to pursue careers in internal medicine, and it may be that AIDS is part of the reason. No other disease in modern times has engendered such frustration, resentment and anxiety or demanded more compassion, intelligence, selflessness and integrity on the part of health professionals.

A disease such as AIDS drains an economy in many ways. AIDS imposes an economic toll on every business, school, public agency, church congregation and community group responsive to the epidemic. In direct costs (those covering medical, scientific and other social expenditures) AIDS will cost the American public tens of billions of dollars over the next decade; indirect costs (such as lost wages from premature death and disability) will add several hundred billion more.

U.S. Public Health Service expenditures on AIDS have grown from approximately $60 million in fiscal 1984 to more than $900 million in fiscal 1988. The budget request for 1989 exceeds $1.2 billion, including $400 million for the Centers for Disease Control and $600 million for the National Institutes of Health. These sums cover scientific research, disease surveillance, prevention and control efforts. Total Federal expenditures for AIDS in fiscal 1989 are projected to exceed $2 billion, including $600 million for the Federal share of patient care through Medicaid.

At the state level, expenditures on AIDS have also risen dramatically, from less than $10 million in 1984 to more than $150 million in 1988. Much of

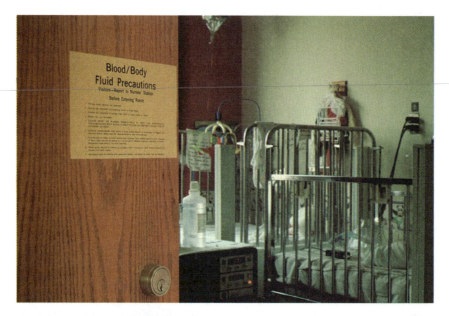

Figure 68 SPECIAL-PRECAUTION SIGNS identify hospital rooms of HIV-positive patients (here children) and remind staff to follow special procedures for handling blood or other fluids. Recently the Centers for Disease Control have recommended that hospitals adopt universal precautions and treat all patients' secretions as if they contained HIV.

that is spent by California and New York; in fiscal 1988 the two states accounted for 46 percent of all AIDS cases and more than 60 percent of state expenditures. On the level of the cities, expenditures are also great: New York City spent more than $130 million on AIDS in 1988 and has budgeted $170 million for the fiscal year 1989, mainly because most of the city's AIDS patients are cared for in public hospitals.

One of the most remarkable and heartening byproducts of the HIV epidemic in the U.S. has been the development of grass-roots organizations dedicated to serving the needs of people with AIDS. An early and sustained commitment to building these organizations has come from the homosexual community. Groups such as the Shanti Project in San Francisco, the Gay Men's Health Crisis, Inc., in New York City and the AIDS Action Committee in Boston were begun in an effort to reach out and relieve the suffering of patients the world seemed to have

turned against. As nonprofit, community-based organizations, they have provided a way for thousands of volunteers to give countless hours of assistance and comfort to patients, their loved ones and families. These organizations developed AIDS telephone hotlines and created specific educational materials for various cultural groups at high risk of HIV infection. They have also been outspoken and effective advocates for all those touched by the epidemic. In a larger social sense, these groups have served as bridges between the gay and lesbian and the straight communities, bringing together individuals who share a commitment to humanitarian goals and a refusal to give in to a lethal enemy.

AIDS has attracted the support of celebrities, business leaders and private foundations. Following the death of her friend Rock Hudson, Elizabeth Taylor became the National Chair of the American Foundation for AIDS Research (AmFAR), the only national foundation dedicated solely to combating

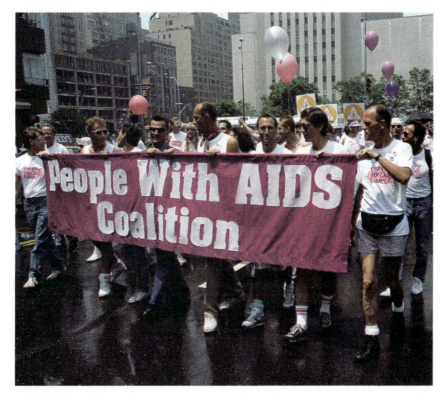

Figure 69 GAY COMMUNITY has fought for increased awareness of AIDS and for greater funding of AIDS-related projects. About 100,000 people marched in New York's Gay Liberation Day parade earlier this year, including the People With AIDS Coalition.

AIDS. AmFAR has raised and devoted millions of dollars to scientific research and has recently broadened its agenda to include innovative educational and community-based service programs.

In 1986 the Robert Wood Johnson Foundation of Princeton, N.J., committed more than $20 million to projects for developing comprehensive and coordinated care for patients with AIDS. More recently the Johnson Foundation has invited applications for support of community-based prevention and service programs. In 1987 the Ford Foundation announced a collaborative, $4.5-million AIDS prevention and service program. By mid-1987 more than 150 foundations were providing support to AIDS-related projects.

Several major insurance companies have spent millions of dollars sponsoring AIDS education programs. Metropolitan Life underwrote the 1987 broadcast of the National AIDS Awareness Test on U.S. television. The New York Life Insurance Co. provided support for the New York City Department of Health's initial advertising campaign to prevent AIDS, a campaign that was developed pro bono by the advertising firm Saatchi & Saatchi Compton, Inc. Scores of prominent individuals in the arts, sports and business communities have lent their time, names and dollars to the struggle against AIDS.

Medical care for those suffering from AIDS is expensive. Estimates of the average lifetime medical costs per patient in the U.S. have ranged from less than $30,000 to more than $140,000, with more recent figures in the vicinity of from $50,000 to $60,000 per patient. These costs do not, of course, include the many thousands of hours that volun-

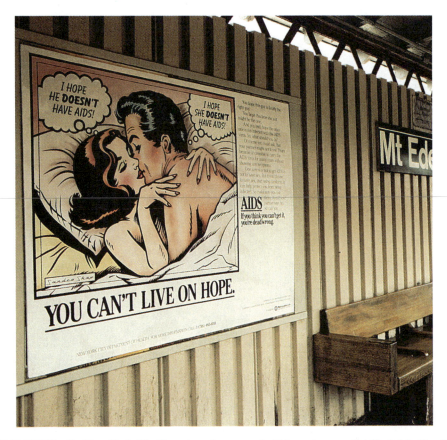

Figure 70 CAMPAIGN by the New York City Department of Health with the help of Saatchi & Saatchi Compton, Inc., is aimed at preventing the spread of AIDS among heterosexuals. This poster was distributed in New York subways in English and Spanish.

teers, family members and friends have contributed to the care of AIDS patients in cities across the U.S. It should be noted that although the cost of treating a patient with AIDS is high, it is well within the range of costs for severely ill patients with other conditions. Patients who require liver transplants, for example, have lifetime medical costs that are three to four times higher on the average than those of an AIDS patient.

Advances in medical care have begun to lower the cost of high-quality services to AIDS patients. The Kaiser-Permanente Medical Group of northern California, for example, established an outpatient center in 1986 to administer various AIDS therapies, including the life-prolonging drug AZT. During its first 18 months of operation the outpatient treatment center saved an estimated 3,500 hospital days. Although pharmacy costs nearly doubled between 1986 and the first half of 1987, average costs for the care of an AIDS patient declined 20 percent because of a 36 percent drop in overall hospital expenses during that period. New treatments in the future may further reduce and possibly eliminate some costs. On the other hand, new and expensive treatment could increase the average cost of care. The uncertain cost of future therapy is another hazy segment in the crystal ball foretelling the future of AIDS.

Total personal medical costs for AIDS will depend both on the average cost per patient and the number of patients. Uncertainty about the future size of the epidemic increases with the distance of the projection. The U.S. Public Health Service recently predicted that 450,000 cases will have been diagnosed by the end of 1993, extending its earlier estimate of 270,000 by the end of 1991. Personal medical costs for AIDS patients during 1991 have been projected to reach levels of between $4.5 and $8.5 billion.

Other costs associated with AIDS patients are subtler. When a hospital adopts universal precautions requiring frequent use of disposable gloves, gowns, masks and protective eyewear, hires additional infectious-disease specialists and infection-control personnel, follows special blood-screening and laboratory procedures and undertakes education and counseling programs for its staff, such costs are spread over all patients and are not found on the bills of those having a diagnosis of AIDS.

The HIV epidemic also results in medical expenditures for patients who are not infected with the virus. The "worried well" who experience general symptoms of fatigue, anxiety or poor appetite may seek medical care and testing because they are concerned about HIV infection. Family members and friends of patients with HIV infection may appropriately seek psychological counseling. HIV infection can also indirectly contribute to the rise of other infections in the community. After declining for many decades, tuberculosis has begun to increase in the U.S. Between 1984 and 1986 reported cases jumped 36 percent in New York City. Today these new cases are found mainly in patients with HIV infection, but as more people in the community develop active tuberculosis the risk of spread to those not infected with HIV will increase. As if to taunt progress in the life sciences in the 20th century, HIV not only has caused the disease most feared in America near the end of the century but also has fueled a resurgence of tuberculosis, the disease most feared at the beginning of the century.

Between 10,000 and 20,000 children in the U.S. are expected to have symptomatic HIV infection in 1991, most of them infected at birth by their mothers. This will represent a 10-to-20-fold increase over the number of newborns afflicted by the end of 1988. In New York City at present between 1 and 2 percent of all women giving birth are infected with HIV, and the proportion rises to more than 5 percent in some areas. The circumstances of life for many of these mothers—poor, ill, unwed and dependent on drugs—prevent them from caring for their infants. Half of the babies may escape infection, yet they have no place to go; many remain in the hospital, where the cost for their care can exceed $250,000 per year. Both the newborns and those who pay their bills would benefit from expanded nursery care outside the hospital, and if the projected number of infected newborns is even remotely correct, the need for many more nonhospital nursery facilities is acute.

The HIV epidemic exposes and exacerbates shortcomings in the system of paying for health care in the U.S. One in five AIDS patients has no insurance; 40 percent of AIDS patients are covered by Medicaid (more than four times the proportion in the general population). Medicaid, a program designed to cover the medical costs of the indigent, is a partnership between the Federal and state governments. Because of the variability in state rules for eligibility, Medicaid covers only 40 percent of those with incomes below the poverty line and frequently pays less than the cost of care. Even private insurers often do not cover the kinds of services—

outpatient, home and hospice care—most needed by people infected with HIV. Private health insurance, for example, generally covers only 15 percent of the cost of drugs prescribed outside the hospital.

These problems can be solved by adopting a number of different strategies: state-based insurance risk pools or subsidies for uninsured patients; reliance on case managers to determine whether insurers should pay for services normally not covered; adjustments in the national standards of Medicaid eligibility and payment; simplification of procedures for states to request flexibility in Medicaid coverage; further extension of insurance coverage for employees who lose their jobs; mandated employer health insurance, and broadened Federal and state support of health insurance. In the case of AIDS, medicine and economy go hand in hand: failure to bring the means of payment into line with patient needs is dime wise and dollar foolish.

Although the costs associated with AIDS are undeniably great, those costs must be put into perspective. The U.S. spends more than half a trillion dollars per year on medical care. Even allowing for a relatively pessimistic projection of the AIDS epidemic, the billions spent on AIDS over the next five years will amount to a small fraction of the country's total health-care expenditures. In the cities and states hardest hit by the epidemic, however, the financial toll will be much heavier. Medical care for the additional cases expected in New York City by 1991 are estimated to cost $100 per resident, in San Francisco $350 per resident.

In parts of Africa and the Caribbean, where HIV infection is more prevalent than in the U.S., weakened economies are much less able to sustain the onslaught of the disease. In the city of Kinshasa in Zaire between 4 and 8 percent of the total population and more than a fourth of the hospitalized patients are thought to be infected with HIV. Many of those infected are in the educated middle class and are business people and professionals. In a dramatic press conference held in October, 1987, the president of Zambia announced that his son had died of AIDS. Demographic projections suggest that the long-term impact of AIDS on these populations may be similar to a prolonged war. In countries where the per capita national product is measured in hundreds of dollars and annual per capita expenditures on health care are $5 or less, a drug such as AZT that costs $8,000 per year might as well be nonexistent.

The World Health Organization's Global Program on AIDS convened an extraordinary World Summit of Ministers of Health in London in January, 1988. Their conference concluded with a declaration on AIDS prevention that emphasized broadening the scope of education, promoting worldwide exchange of information and reinforcing the importance of nondiscriminatory policies. The 41st World Health Assembly in Geneva in May adopted a formal resolution endorsing confidentiality of HIV testing and urging member states to avoid discrimination against AIDS patients in the provision of services, in employment and in travel. A similar call for antidiscrimination laws was the first recommendation of the June 1988 report of the U.S. Presidential Commission on the HIV Epidemic.

Public-health officials should have three primary objectives in coping with the AIDS epidemic. They are, first, to provide compassionate, effective and cost-sensitive care to the people who have the disease; second, to prevent further transmission of the disease, and third, to aggressively pursue scientific research that may lead to more effective prevention, diagnosis and treatment. The first objective requires committed and well-trained health professionals, increased services and a responsive health-care financing system. The second requires a sustained and unprecedented educational effort, judicious use of available public-health measures and special attention to minority communities, intravenous drug users and other populations at high risk of infection. The third requires building new human and institutional capacities, balancing basic and applied objectives and designing coherent research plans.

A strategy to accomplish these objectives stands on four cornerstones. The first is leadership that will inspire, direct and organize the fight against AIDS at local, state, national and international levels. The second is adequate financial resources to do the job, drawn mostly from public sources but also from some private ones. The third is legal protection against discrimination, on which so much else depends. And the fourth is an accurate and timely surveillance system that can track and project the status of the epidemic. The future course of the HIV epidemic is uncertain and a strategy that takes account of such uncertainty is imperative.

Our world has been made a different place by the human immunodeficiency virus. More profoundly, our society is being shaped by our response to the epidemic. Will AIDS enhance understanding and tolerance of different sexual orientations, or will it harden traditional norms of acceptable and deviant sexual behavior? Will AIDS be perceived as a universal threat to all humanity, or will it be regarded as a problem of the underclass, the poor and uneducated, and the minorities? Will AIDS heighten the tension between moralistic and pragmatic approaches to behavior and health, or can solutions be found that are both effective and morally acceptable? Will AIDS evoke the selfless dedication of physicians, nurses and other health professionals, or will caregivers shun AIDS patients and seek other ways to practice their craft? How we choose to answer such questions, and the society we thus shape, is up to us.

Epilogue

AIDS: An unknown distance still to go

. . .

Lewis Thomas

In a long lifetime of looking at biomedical research, I have never seen anything to touch the progress that has already been made in laboratories working on the AIDS virus. Considering that the disease was recognized only seven years ago and that its agent, HIV, is one of the most complex and baffling organisms on earth, the achievement is an astonishment.

If AIDS had first appeared 10 or 15 years ago, before the research technologies of molecular biology had developed the marvelous tool of recombinant DNA, we would still be completely stuck, quite unable even to make intelligent guesses about the cause of the disease. Thanks to the new methods, which emerged from entirely basic research having nothing at all to do with any medical problem, we now know more about HIV's structure, molecular composition, behavior and target cells than about those of any other virus in the world. The work, in short, is going well. But it is in its early stages, and there is an unknown distance still to go. At the moment three lines of research seem to me to hold the most promise, and already there is a conspicuous shortfall in the funds needed for each of them.

One approach, the most direct of the three but perhaps the most difficult and unpredictable, is in the field of pharmacology. We need a new class of antiviral drugs capable of killing off viruses inside the cells they invade, without killing the cells themselves. These drugs must be comparable in effectiveness to the antibiotics that began to be deployed against bacterial infections 50 years ago. There are a few partially active drugs that may turn out to be the primitive precursors of such a class, but their effectiveness is still incomplete, they are temporarily palliative at best and their toxicity is unacceptable. However, there are no theoretical barriers to the development of decisively effective antivirals, including drugs to stop the replication of retroviruses such as HIV. What is urgently required—is indispensable, in fact—is some new and very deep information about the intimate details of retroviruses and the enzyme systems that enable them to penetrate and multiply within the target cells that are their specialty.

Second, we need an abundance of new information about how the human immune system can neutralize HIV. Even if and when an antiviral drug is in hand that really works to control infection in individual cases, the only imaginable way to prevent the continuing spread of HIV will be by means of a vaccine. The design of a vaccine calls for better understanding of the molecular labels at the surface of the virus and knowledge of which among these labels represents a point of vulnerability for an immune response. Since this particular virus has the strange property of changing its labels from time to time—even at different stages of the disease in the same patient—this will be no easy task. A few vaccine trials are already under way in small cohorts of human subjects. There is no reason to be optimistic about these at the present time, nor is there any way to hurry things up. With a lot of luck, some laboratory may succeed in identifying a stable and genuinely vulnerable target molecule in HIV, and then a vaccine will be feasible.

A third line of research involves the human immune system itself, the primary victim of HIV. Most, if not all, patients with AIDS die from other kinds of infection rather than from any direct, lethal action of the virus itself. The process is a subtle one, something like an end game in chess. What the virus does, selectively and with exquisite precision, is to take out the population of lymphocytes responsible for defending the body against all sorts of microbes in the world outside, most of which are harmless to healthy human beings. In a sense, the patients are not dying because of the HIV virus; they are being killed by great numbers of other bacteria and viruses that can now swarm into a defenseless host. Research is needed to gain a deeper understanding of the biology of the immune cells, in the hope of preserving them or replacing them by transplanting normal immune cells. This may be necessary even if viricidal drugs are developed: by the time such drugs destroy the virus in some patients, the immune system may already have been wiped out, and the only open course will be to replace it.

This third line of investigation had become one of the liveliest fields in basic immunology long before the appearance of AIDS, and what is now needed is an intensification of the research. In my own view (perhaps biased because of my background in immunology), it is the most urgent and potentially promising of all current approaches to the AIDS problem.

To sum up, AIDS is a scientific research problem, to be solved only by basic investigation in good laboratories. The research done in the past few years has been elegant and highly productive, with results that tell us one sure thing: AIDS is a soluble problem, albeit an especially complex and difficult one. No one can predict at this stage how it will turn out or where the really decisive answers will be found, but the possibilities are abundant and the prospects are bright.

It is particularly encouraging that the basic research most needed is becoming conducted by collaborative groups in both academic and industrial establishments. That is a new phenomenon in this country, well worth noting in the present context. Until just recently—the past decade or so—the university laboratories and their counterparts in the pharmaceutical industry tended to hold apart from each other, indeed rather looked down their noses at each other. It took the biological revolution of the 1970's, and specifically the new technologies of recombinant DNA and monoclonal antibodies, to bring scientists from both communities into a close intellectual relation. Now the lines we used to think of as separating basic and applied research into two distinct categories have become more and more blurred. Academic and industrial scientists recognize that they are in the same line of work, and research partnerships are being set up all over the place.

I take this to be an exceedingly healthy transformation in our institutions. One response to the development will have to be the recruiting and training of more bright young people for the work ahead. As an academic, I am delighted to see so many university scientists eyeing new horizons and thinking of career possibilities in industry. It is a good sign for the future of this country in our competition with others in pharmaceutical science, and a good sign as well for the solution of the AIDS problem.

The Authors

ROBERT C. GALLO and **LUC MONTAGNIER** ("The AIDS Epidemic") are the investigators who established the cause of AIDS. Gallo is chief of the Laboratory of Tumor Cell Biology at the National Cancer Institute. Montagnier is professor of virology at the Pasteur Institute in Paris and director of research at the French National Center for Scientific Research (CNRS).

WILLIAM A. HASELTINE and **FLOSSIE WONG-STAAL** ("The Molecular Biology of the AIDS Virus"). Haseltine holds appointments at the Dana-Farber Cancer Institute, the Harvard Medical School and the Harvard School of Public Health. He received his doctorate in biophysics from Harvard and became interested in retroviruses in 1972 as a postdoctoral student at the Massachusetts Institute of Technology. Haseltine's current research concerns retroviruses in leukemia, disorders of the central nervous system and AIDS. Wong-Staal is head of the section on the molecular genetics of hematopoietic cells at the National Cancer Institute. She holds a Ph.D. in molecular biology from the University of California at Los Angeles. After joining the NCI in 1973, she became interested in the role of retroviruses and oncogenes in disease—an interest she pursued as the first human retroviruses were discovered.

MAX ESSEX and **PHYLLIS J. KANKI** ("The Origins of the AIDS Virus") work together at the Harvard School of Public Health, where he heads the department of cancer biology and is chairman of the Harvard AIDS Institute and she is a research scientist in the institute. Essex has a doctor's degree in veterinary medicine from Michigan State University and a Ph.D. from the University of California at Davis. His laboratory discovered the human-retrovirus envelope proteins, which are major candidates for future AIDS vaccines. In 1986 Essex shared the Lasker Award in clinical medical research with Robert C. Gallo and Luc Montagnier. Kanki has a doctor's degree in veterinary medicine from the University of Minnesota and a D.Sc. from the Harvard School of Public Health. After working at the New England Regional Primate Research Center, she joined Essex' laboratory in 1983. Kanki is currently leading an investigation of the biology of HIV-2 in West Africa.

WILLIAM L. HEYWARD and **JAMES W. CURRAN** ("The Epidemiology of AIDS in the U.S.") are colleagues in the AIDS Program at the Centers for Disease Control (CDC) in Atlanta. Heyward is chief of international activities for the program. He was working in a CDC laboratory in Alaska in 1985 when the first AIDS case was diagnosed in that state. Since then his involvement in AIDS research has increased steadily; he moved to Atlanta in 1987. Curran is director of the AIDS Program. He was a member of the CDC task force that was organized after the first AIDS cases were diagnosed in 1981 to help make investigators aware of the disease and to stimulate the research that led to the discovery of its cause. The authors would like to note that the photographs accompanying their chapter were not provided by the CDC.

JONATHAN M. MANN, JAMES CHIN, PETER PIOT and **THOMAS QUINN** ("The International Epidemiology of AIDS") collaborate on the investigation of AIDS. Mann has been director of the World Health Organization's Global AIDS Program (GPA) since its inception in 1986. Chin is chief of the AIDS Surveillance Unit for the GPA. Piot is professor of microbiology at the Institute of Tropical Medicine in Antwerp. Quinn is on the medical staff of the National Institutes of Health and at the Johns Hopkins Hospital in Baltimore.

ROBERT R. REDFIELD and **DONALD S. BURKE** ("HIV Infection: The Clinical Picture") are colleagues at the Walter Reed Army Institute of Research in Washington, D.C. Redfield is chief of the section of retrovirology, immunoregulation and immunotherapy and medical director of the clinical virology laboratory. He was given the first annual Thomas Parran Award for his work on HIV infection. Burke is a colonel in the Medical Corps of the U.S. Army. He has been chief of the Department of Virus Diseases at the Institute of Research since 1984.

JOHATHAN N. WEBER and **ROBIN A. WEISS** ("HIV Infection: The Cellular Picture") have been working together since 1985, when Weber joined Weiss's laboratory to get training in virology. Weber is a senior lecturer in infectious disease at the Royal Postgraduate Medical School at Hammersmith Hospital in London. He took his undergraduate degree in archaeology and anthropology at the University of Cambridge and his M.D. at St. Bartholomew's Hospital Medical College in London. He is coeditor of *International AIDS Journal*. Weiss is director of the Institute for Cancer Research in London. He studied at the University of London, where he was awarded a Ph.D. in zoology in 1969. He has been interested in retroviruses since the beginning of his research career; his early work concerned the transmission of retroviruses in chickens, including the Mendelian inheritance of viral genes. In recent years Weiss has concentrated on the retroviruses that cause leukemia and AIDS, with particular attention to their cellular receptors.

ROBERT YARCHOAN, HIROAKI MITSUYA and **SAMUEL BRODER** ("AIDS Therapies") are in the Clinical Oncology Program of the National Cancer Institute (NCI). In 1984 they began searching for antiretroviral AIDS therapies. Yarchoan, a senior investigator, earned his M.D. from the University of Pennsylvania in 1975. He joined the NCI in 1978, where he specialized in viral immunology and later focused on AIDS. Mitsuya received an M.D. in 1975 and a Doctor of Medical Science degree in 1982 from the Kumamoto University Medical School in Japan. He joined the NCI in 1982, where he developed the assay system used to find the anti-HIV activity of dideoxynucleosides. Broder, who is head of the program, received his M.D. in 1970 from the University of Michigan. He joined the NCI in 1972. He was among the first to identify antiviral drugs that could be moved quickly from the test tube into AIDS patients.

THOMAS J. MATTHEWS and **DANI P. BOLOGNESI** ("AIDS Vaccines") work together in the surgical virology laboratory at the Duke University Medical Center, where they have been researching AIDS vaccines for the past four years. Matthews got his Ph.D. from the University of Missouri in 1967 and held a postdoctoral appointment at the University of Wisconsin at Madison before going to Duke in 1977. Matthews is a member of the National Cancer Institute's AIDS Vaccine Task Force. Bolognesi got his Ph.D. from Duke in 1967 and has been on the faculty there since 1971. He is a consultant for the National Institutes of Health AIDS Executive Committee and a member of the scientific advisory committee of the American Foundation for AIDS Research.

HARVEY V. FINEBERG ("The Social Dimensions of AIDS") is dean of the Harvard School of Public Health. He is interested in medical and governmental decision making and has helped to set Government policy with respect to the AIDS epidemic. He was a member of the National Academy of Sciences/Institute of Medicine committee that published the 1986 report *Confronting AIDS*. Fineberg is a three-time Harvard University alumnus, having received his B.A., M.D. and Ph.D. degrees there.

LEWIS THOMAS ("AIDS: An Unknown Distance Still to Go") is president emeritus of the Memorial Sloan-Kettering Cancer Center and scholar in residence at the Cornell University Medical College.

Bibliographies

1. The AIDS Epidemic

Barré-Sinoussi, F., et al. 1983. Isolation of the T-lymphotropic retrovirus from a patient at risk for acquired immune deficiency syndrome (AIDS). *Science* 220 (May 20): 868–871.

Clavel, François, et al. 1986. Isolation of a new human retrovirus from West African patients with AIDS. *Science* 233 (July 18): 343–346.

Gallo, Robert C. 1986. The first human retrovirus. *Scientific American* 255 (December): 78–88.

———. 1987. The AIDS virus. *Scientific American* 256 (January): 38–48.

1987. Commentary: The chronology of AIDS research. *Nature* 326 (April 2): 435–436.

2. The Molecular Biology of the Aids Virus

Haseltine, William A., Ernest F. Terwilliger, Craig A. Rosen and Joseph G. Sodroski. 1988. Structure and function of human pathogenic retroviruses. In *Retrovirus biology: An emerging role in human diseases*, eds. Robert C. Gallo and Flossie Wong-Staal. Marcel Dekker, Inc.

Rappoport, Jay, and Flossie Wong-Staal. 1988. *Cis-* and *trans*-activation of HIV. In *Concepts of viral pathogenesis*, eds. Abner Notkins and Michael Oldstone. Springer-Verlag.

Franza, B. Robert, Jr., Bryan R. Cullen and Flossie Wong-Staal, eds. 1988. *The control of human retrovirus gene expression*. Cold Spring Harbor Laboratory.

3. The Origins of the AIDS Virus

Kanki, P. J., M. F. McLane, N. W. King, Jr., N. L. Letvin, R. D. Hunt, P. Sehgal, M. D. Daniel, R. C. Desrosiers and M. Essex. 1985. Serologic identification and characterization of a macaque T-lymphotropic retrovirus closely related to human HTLV-III. *Science* 228 (June 7): 1199–1201.

Kanki, P. J., J. Alroy and M. Essex. 1985. Isolation of T-lymphotropic retrovirus related to HTLV-III/LAV from wild-caught African green monkeys. *Science* 230 (November 22): 951–954.

Barin, F., S. M'Boup, F. Denis, P. Kanki, J. S. Allan, T. H. Lee and M. Essex. 1985. Serologic evidence for virus related to simian T-lymphotropic retrovirus III in residents of West Africa. *The Lancet* 2 (December 21/28): 1387–1389.

Kanki, Phyllis J., et al. 1987. Human T-lymphotropic virus type 4 and the human immunodeficiency virus in West Africa. *Science* 236 (May 15): 827–831.

Marlink, Richard G., et al. 1988. Clinical, hematologic, and immunologic cross-sectional evaluation of individuals exposed to human immunodeficiency virus type-2 (HIV-2). *AIDS research and human retroviruses* 4 (April): 137–148.

4. The Epidemiology of AIDS in the U.S.

Cole, Helene M., and George D. Lundberg, eds. 1986. *AIDS: From the beginning.* American Medical Association.

Wormser, Gary P., Rosalyn E. Stahl and Edward J. Bottone. 1987. *AIDS (acquired immunodeficiency syndrome) and other manifestations of HIV infection.* Noyes Publications.

Dondero, Timothy J., and the HIV Data Analysis Team. 1987. Human immunodeficiency virus infection in the United States: A review of current knowledge. *MMWR (Morbidity and Mortality Weekly Report)* 36 (Supplement No. S-6).

1988. *Report of the presidential commission on the human immunodeficiency virus epidemic.* U.S. Government Printing Office.

5. The International Epidemiology of Aids

Widdus, Roy, ed. 1986. *Confronting AIDS: Directions for public health, health care, and research.* National Academy Press.

1987. AIDS—A global perspective. *The Western Journal of Medicine* 147 (December).

Weiss, Robin, ed. 1988. *Confronting AIDS: Update 1988.* National Academy Press.

1988. The AIDS issue. *Science* 239 (February 5).

6. HIV Infection: The Clinical Picture

Redfield, Robert R., D. Craig Wright and Edmund C. Tramont. 1986. The Walter Reed staging classification for HTLV-III/LAV infection. *The New England Journal of Medicine* 314 (January 9): 131–132.

Redfield, Robert R., and Donald S. Burke. 1987. Shadow on the land: HIV infection. *Viral Immunology* 1 (Spring): 69–81.

Price, Richard W., Bruce Brew, John Sidtis, Marc Rosenblum, Adrienne C. Scheck and Paul Cleary. 1988. The brain in AIDS: Central nervous system HIV-1 infection and AIDS dementia complex. *Science* 239 (February 5): 586–592.

Glatt, Aaron E., Keith Chirgwin and Sheldon H. Landesman. 1988. Treatment of infections associated with human immunodeficiency virus. *The New England Journal of Medicine* 318 (June 2): 1439–1448.

7. HIV Infection: The Cellular Picture

Dalgleish, Angus G., Peter C. L. Beverley, Paul R. Clapman, Dorothy H. Crawford, Melvyn F. Greaves and Robin A. Weiss. 1984. The CD4 (T4) antigen is an essential component of the receptor for the AIDS retrovirus. *Nature* 312 (December 20–27): 763–767.

Maddon, Paul Jay. Angus G. Dalgleish, J. Steven McDougal, Paul R. Clapham, Robin A. Weiss and Richard Axel. 1986. The T4 gene encodes the AIDS virus receptor and is expressed in the immune system and the brain. *Cell* 47 (November 7): 333–348.

Peterson, Andrew, and Brian Seed. 1988. Genetic analysis of monoclonal antibody and HIV binding sites on the human lymphocyte antigen CD4. *Cell* 54 (July 1): 65–72.

8. AIDS Therapies

Broder, Samuel, ed. 1987. *AIDS: Modern concepts and therapeutic challenges.* Marcel Dekker, Inc.

Yarchoan, Robert, and Samuel Broder. 1987. Development of antiretroviral therapy for the acquired immunodeficiency syndrome and related disorders: A progress report. *The New England Journal of Medicine* 316 (February 26): 557–564.

Mitsuya, Hiroaki, and Samuel Broder. 1987. Strategies for antiviral therapy in AIDS. *Nature* 325 (February 26): 773–778.

Fischl, Margaret A., et al. 1987. The efficacy of azidothymidine (AZT) in the treatment of patients with AIDS and AIDS-related complex: A double-blind, placebo-controlled trial. *The New England Journal of Medicine* 317 (July 23): 185–191.

Smith, Douglas H., Randal A. Byrn, Scot A. Marsters, Timothy Gregory, Jerome E. Groopman and Daniel J. Capon. 1987. Blocking of HIV-1 infectivity by a soluble, secreted form of the CD4 antigen. *Science* 238 (December 18): 1704–1707.

9. AIDS Vaccines

McNeill, William H. 1976. *Plagues and peoples.* Doubleday & Co.

Hilleman, Maurice R. 1984. Whither immunization against viral infections? *Annals of Internal Medicine* 101 (December): 852–858.

———. 1987. Prospects for a vaccine to protect against AIDS. In *Viral hepatitis and AIDS*, ed. Victor M. Villarejos. Editorial Trejos Hermanos (San José, Costa Rica).

Bolognesi, Dani P. 1988. Natural immunity to HIV and its possible relationship to vaccine strategies. *Microbiological Sciences* 5 (August): 236–241.

10. The Social Dimensions of AIDS

Widdus, Roy, ed. 1986. *Confronting AIDS: Directions for public health, health care, and research*. National Academy Press.
World Summit of Ministers of Health on Programmes for AIDS Prevention. 1988. *AIDS prevention and control*. Pergamon Press.

Weiss, Robin, ed. 1988. *Confronting AIDS: Update 1988*. National Academy Press.
Fineberg, Harvey V. 1988. Education to prevent AIDS: Prospects and obstacles. *Science* 239 (February 5): 592–596.
1988. *Report of the presidential commission on the human immunodeficiency virus epidemic*. U.S. Government Printing Office.

INDEX

Page numbers in *italics* indicate illustrations.

Abortion
  prevention of AIDS, 60
Abrams, Donald I., 91
Acquired immune
    deficiency syndrome
    (AIDS)
  anti-idiotype therapy,
    83–84
  blood tests, 11
  causes of, 4, 7
  discovery of, 1
  economic costs, 116–117
  identification of, 63–64
  international
    epidemiology, 51–61
  molecular biology of,
    13–25
  mutations, 24
  origins of, 2, 27–37
  prevention of, 114–115
  reported cases, *41, 55, 56*
  social dimensions of,
    111–121
  therapies, 10, 83, 119
  U.S. epidemiology, 39–49
  vaccines, 10, 101–110
  virus particles, *1*
  West Africa, 34–36, *36*
  (*See also* human
    immunodeficiency
    virus)
Acyclovir, 69, 95, 99
Adenosine, 92, *93*
Adult *T*-cell leukemia
    (ATL), 2
Advertising
  AIDS education
    campaigns, 118
Africa
  AIDS epidemiology, 7, 9,
    51, 52–55, 114
  AIDS prevention, 11
  blood screening, 60
  economic losses from
    AIDS, 59, 120
  HIV infection, 30, 45, 58
  HIV-2 distribution, 35
  HTLV origins, 28
  LAV viruses, 4
  SIV-related viruses, 33–34
  survival time of AIDS
    patients, 52
Africa, central
  AIDS epidemiology, 7, 9,
    53
  AIDS prevention, 11
  AIDS transmission, 41
  HIV infection rate, 30, 45
  HIV infection spread, 37
  SIV-related viruses, 33
African green monkeys
  SIV infection, 27, 30–32,
    34
  STLV infection, 28

African macaque monkeys
  SIV infection, 34
African Old World monkeys
  STLV infection, 28
Age distribution
  U.S. AIDS patients, *46*
AIDS (*see* acquired immune
    deficiency syndrome)
AIDS Action Committee, 117
AIDS dementia, 69–70, 97
AIDS-related complex
    (ARC), 65
Alpha-interferon, 96, *98*, 99
Alum, 107
American Foundation for
    AIDS Research
    (AmFAR), 117–118
Ampligen, *98*, 99
Anal intercourse
  HIV infection risk, 45
Anemia
  AZT therapy, 97
Anergy, 68, *69*
Antibodies, 102
  AIDS vaccines, 108
  blocking infection, *107*
  HIV infection, 105, 106
  HIV therapies, 89–90
Antigen-presenting cells, 80
Antigens
  infection and vaccines, 102
Anti-idiotype antibodies,
    83–84, 90
  AIDS vaccines, 108, *109*
  HIV therapies, 89
Antisense oligonucleotides,
    88, 94–95
Antisense
    phosphorothioates, 95
Apes
  HIV infection, 82
  HIV-related viruses, 27
ARC (*see* AIDS-related
    complex)
Argentina
  AIDS cases, *59*
Asia
  AIDS epidemiology, 53,
    55–56
Asian macaque monkeys
  HIV-related viruses, 30
  simian AIDS, *37*
  SIV infection, 30, 32
  STLV infection, 28
ATL (*see* adult *T*-cell
    leukemia)
Australia
  AIDS epidemiology, 52,
    53, 55, *59*
Austria
  AIDS cases, *59*
Autoimmune response, 9
  AIDS vaccines, 105
Axel, Richard, 76–77

Azidothymidine (AZT or
    3'-azido-2', 3'-dide-
    oxythmidine), 10, 63,
    85, *88*, 92, 96–99
  cost of, 120
  outpatient treatment for
    AIDS, 119
Azidothymidine
    triphosphate, 92

B cells, 80, 102
  herpes infections, 9–10
  HIV infection, 64
  hyperactivity in HIV
    infection, 67, 70
  immune response to
    infection, *105*
Baboons
  SIV infection, 30
Bacteria
  therapeutic agents, 85–87
Bahamas
  AIDS cases, *59*
Baltimore, David, 2, 95
Bangkok, Thailand
  HIV infection and drug
    use, 56
Barin, Francis, 33
Barré-Sinoussi, Françoise, 3
Basel Institute for
    Immunology, 90
Becton Dickinson
    Monoclonal Center,
    Inc., 108
Behavior
  AIDS prevention, 114
Belgium
  AIDS cases, *59*
Berg, G., 87
0.5-β, 89
Beverley, Peter C. L.,
    81–82, 84, 89
Biogen N.V., 90
Bisexuals
  AIDS epidemiology, 41, 52
  transmission of AIDS, 114
Blacks
  AIDS cases, 39, 43, *44*,
    114, 115
Blindness
  and AIDS, 68, 69
Blood and blood products
  AIDS international
    epidemiology, 53, 55
  hospital handling
    procedures, *116*
  screening of donations, 42
  spread of AIDS, 114
  transmission of HIV, 4, 9,
    10, 52
Blood-brain barrier
  HIV infection, 85
Blood tests
  preventing AIDS, 10, 11

Blood transfusions
  AIDS epidemiology, 2,
    41, 42, 45–46, 48, 52,
    54, 60
Bone marrow
  AZT therapy, 97
  HIV infection, 13, 22
Boston, Massachusetts
  AIDS Action Committee,
    117
  AIDS prevention
    programs, 114
Brain
  HIV infection, 69, 80
  HIV therapies, 96–97
Brazil
  AIDS epidemiology, 57,
    59
Breast-feeding
  HIV transmission, 46
Broder, Samuel, 87, 91
Brookmeyer, Ronald, 48
Brunetti, A., 87
Burk family, *63*
Burkina Faso
  HIV infection, 37
Burroughs Wellcome, 92
Burundi
  AIDS cases, *59*
Butare, Rwanda
  AIDS cases, 54

California
  AIDS epidemiology, 40
  AIDS expenditures, 117
Canada
  AIDS epidemiology, 52,
    58, *59*
Cancer
  HIV infection, 65, 70
  Kaposi's sarcoma, 40, 64,
    70, 85
  lymphoid, 28
  retroviral genes, 103
  and retroviruses, 2, 3
  (*See also* leukemia)
CAR sequence (*see*
    cis-acting *rev*-
    responsive sequence)
Caribbean
  AIDS epidemiology, 52,
    53, 57, 114
  economic losses from
    AIDS, 120
Case-control study
  of AIDS, 40
Castanospermine, 96, *98*
Cats
  retroviruses in, 109
CD4, 6–7, 9
  AIDS therapy, 10
  AIDS vaccines, *109*
  antibodies, 105, 108

HIV infection, 22, 37, 64, 65, *66*, 75–84, *88*, 106, *107*
CD4, soluble, 89–91, *98*
Cell death
  HIV infection, 22–23, 65, 80
Cell-mediated response to infection, 102, *105*
Centers for Disease Control, U.S. (CDC), 51, 64
  AIDS epidemiology, 40
  AIDS expenditures, 116
  state programs for HIV, 115
Central Africa (*see* Africa, central)
Central nervous system
  cell death, 23
  HIV infection, 13, 65, 67, 85, 102
Chain termination
  HIV therapies, 92
Chancroid, 54
Cheng-Mayer, Cecilia, 80
Chermann, Jean-Claude, 3
Childbearing
  prevention of AIDS, 60
Childhood leukemia, 99
Children
  AIDS cases, 42–43, 44, 46, 119
  AIDS therapies, 97
  hospital care of AIDS patients, 115
  mortality from AIDS in Africa, 54
  transmission of HIV from mothers, 2, 10, 43, 46, 52
Chile
  AIDS cases, *59*
Chimeric molecules
  HIV therapies, 90
Chimpanzees
  HIV infection, 32, 108
  SIV infection, 30
  STLV infection, 28
China
  AIDS epidemiology, 55
Chiron Corporation, 107
Chromaffin cells
  HIV infection, 80, *81*
Ciba-Geigy AG, 107
Circumcision, female
  spread of HIV, 54
cis-acting repression sequence (CRS), 18, 19, *21*, 23
cis-acting *rev*-responsive sequence (CAR), 18, 19, *21*, 23
Clapham, Paul R., 76, 77
Class II Major Histocompatibility Complex (MHC), 80, 83
Clavel, François, 34
Cognitive function
  HIV infection, 69
Cohen, Jack C., 95
Columbia University, 90
Competitive inhibition
  HIV therapies, 92

Condoms
  prevention of AIDS, 60, 114
Congo
  AIDS epidemiology, 51, 53
Contagion
  fear of, *113*
Contraception
  prevention of AIDS, 60
Core proteins
  HIV, *36*
  SIV, *31*, *34*, *36*
Counseling
  AIDS education, 49
  of HIV-infected people, 60
Cows
  retroviruses, 109
Cross-reactive epitopes, 28, 30
Cross-reactivity of viruses, 28, *31*
CRS sequence (*see cis*-acting repression sequence)
Cryptococcal meningitis, 69
Cryptococcosis, 68
Cryptosporidiosis, chronic, 68
Cytidine, 92
Cytokines
  HIV infection, 64, 65, 69, 70
Cytomegalovirus, 68, 69
Cytosine, *93*
Cytotoxic lymphocytes (*see T* cells, killer)

Dakar
  HIV infection, 36
Dalgleish, Angus G., 76, 77, 84, 108
Dana-Farber Cancer Institute, 90
Daniel, Muthiah D., 30
Dapsone, 69
Darby, Graham K., 92
ddA (*see* 2', 3'-dideoxyadenosine)
ddC (*see* 2', 3'-dideoxycytidine)
ddI (*see* 2', 3'-dideoxyinosine)
De Clerq, Eric, 87
Delayed hypersensitivity
  HIV infection, 68, *69*
Dementia (*see* AIDS dementia; HIV-induced dementia)
Denmark
  AIDS epidemiology, 57, *59*
Desrosiers, Ronald C., 7, 30
Dextran sulfate, 91, *98*, 99
Diagnosis of HIV, 63, 65–67
2',3'-dideoxyadenosine (ddA), 92, 97, 98
Dideoxyadenosine triphosphate, 97
2',3'-dideoxycytidine (ddC), 10, 97, *98*
2',3'-dideoxyinosine (ddI), 92, 97, *98*

Dideoxynucleosides, *88*
  HIV therapies, 92–94, 97
2',3'-dideoxythymidine, 92
Diffuse, undifferentiated non-Hodgkin's lymphoma, 40
Direct-fusion mechanism, 78
Discrimination
  AIDS victims, 120
DNA, viral, 1–2, 4, 14, *15*
  deoxynucleosides, 92, *93*
  genetic regulation, 17
  HIV infection, *18*, 22, 64, 80, 87–*88*
  HIV therapies, 91–92, 94, 95
  mutations and cell replication, 24
DNA probes, 7
Doctors
  care of AIDS patients, 116
Dominican Republic
  AIDS epidemiology, 57–58, *59*
Dreesman, Gordon R., 84
Drug therapies
  for AIDS, 85–99
Drug users, intravenous
  and AIDS in children, 43
  AIDS international epidemiology, 52–55, 56–58, 60
  AIDS U.S. epidemiology, 39, 41, 42, *44*
  blacks and Hispanic AIDS cases, 43
  counseling about AIDS, 49
  HIV infection rate, 45
  public-health measures, 120
  spread of AIDS, 10–11, *113*, 114, 115
Duke University Medical Center, 96

Eastern Europe
  AIDS epidemiology, 53, 57
Economic costs
  AIDS epidemic, 116–117
Education
  AIDS programs, 60
  prevention of AIDS, 10–11, 114
  world information exchange on AIDS, 120
Endogenous viruses, 32
Endosomes
  HIV infection, 77–78
Engleman, Edgar G., 89
env gene, *18*, *36*
Envelope proteins
  AIDS and HIV vaccines, 105, 106
  HIV infection, 14, *16*, 17, 22, 24, 33–34, 75, 79, 82, *101*
  HIV and SIV genetic organization, *36*
  HIV therapies, 89, 91
  SIV, 30, *31*
  VSV (HIV), 76

Enzymes
  HIV and SIV genetic organization, *36*
  HIV therapies, 94–96
  reverse transcriptase, 2
  viral genetic information, 14
  virion assembly, *16*
Epidemiology of AIDS, 6
  international, 51–61
  U.S., 39–49
Essex, Max, 2, 4, 9
Ethiopia
  AIDS cases, *59*
Europe
  AIDS epidemiology, 56–57
  HIV infection estimates, 58
  HIV infection rate, 30
Exogenous viruses, 32

Fansidar, 69
Fatalities
  AIDS patients, *41*, 52
Feline leukemia (FeLV), 2, 103
Fischl, Margaret A., 96
Food and Drug Administration, U.S.
  AZT, 96
Ford Foundation, 118
Forecasting
  AIDS trends, 47–48, 58, 120
France
  AIDS blood test, 11
  AIDS cases, *59*
  AIDS vaccines, 110
Franco-American AIDS Foundation, 11
French Guiana
  AIDS cases, *59*
Furmanski, Philip, 87
Fusion factor
  HIV infection, 22

gag gene, *18*, *36*
Gallo, Robert C., 2–4, 6, 7, 9, 27, 28, 87, 106, 110
Ganciclovir, 69
Gartner, Suzanne, 6
Gay Liberation Day parade, *117*
Gay Men's Health Crisis, Inc., 117
Gelderblom, Hans, 3, 13, *17*
Genentech Inc., 90
Genes, regulatory
  HIV, 15–17, *18*, *20*
Genes, viral
  cell death, 23
  HIV, 18–22
  HIV therapies, 95
Genital herpes
  HIV infection, 45
Geographical distribution of AIDS, 53
  United States, 114
Germany
  AIDS vaccines, 110
Glial cells
  HIV infection, 80, *81*

Global Program on AIDS (GPA), 51, 58, 59–61, 120
Gluckman, Jean-Claude, 3
Glycoproteins, 106
  HIV, 87
  HIV therapies, 89, 91
  (See also envelope proteins; gp41; gp120; gp160)
Glycosylation, 96
Goldstein, Allan L., 108
Gonnorrhea
  decline of, 48
Gottleib, Michael S., 76
gp41, 4, 14, 106
  HIV infection, 22, 79, 107
  HIV therapies, 91
gp120, 4, 9, 14
  AIDS vaccines, 103–105, 106
  HIV infection, 64–66, 75–78, 79, 81–84, 88, 107
  HIV therapies, 89, 90
  SIV, 31
  viral growth, 22
gp160, 106
  AIDS vaccine, 106–107, 108
  SIV, 31
Great Britain
  AIDS vaccines, 110
Greece
  AIDS cases, 59
Gruter, Robert, 96
Guanosine, 92
Guinea-Bissau, West Africa
  AIDS infection, 7
Gut cells
  HIV infection, 80

H9 cell, 11
Haase, Ashley T., 105
Hahn, Beatrice H., 6
Hairy-cell leukemia, 2
Haiti
  AIDS epidemiology, 41, 57–58, 59
  HIV infection rate, 45
  survival time of AIDS patients, 52
Harvard Institute of International Development, 58
Haseltine, William A., 4, 82, 89, 96
Haynes, Barton F., 106
HBLV (see human B-cell lymphotropic virus)
Health-care workers
  care of AIDS patients, 115–116
  risk of HIV infection, 45
HeLa cells, 76–77
Hemophiliacs
  AIDS epidemiology in U.S., 39, 41–43, 48
  LAV viruses, 4
Hepatitis B vaccine, 103, 105
Herpes simplex virus, 68, 69
Herpes viruses, 9–10
  HIV replication, 95

Heterosexuals
  AIDS education, 118
  AIDS epidemiology, 42, 44, 52, 53, 54, 57
  HIV transmission, 7, 41, 45
HGP-30, 108
HHV-6 (see human herpes virus 6)
Hilleman, Maurice R., 110
Hirsch, Martin S., 96
Hispanics
  AIDS epidemiology, 39, 43, 44, 114, 115
Histoplasmosis
  and AIDS, 68, 69
HIV (see human immunodeficiency virus)
HIVAC (HIV vaccine) group, 110
HIV-induced dementia, 87
  (See also AIDS dementia)
Hockley, David, 75
Homosexuals
  AIDS epidemiology in U.S., 39–45, 48
  AIDS international epidemiology, 52–54, 56–58
  diagnosis of AIDS, 2
  LAV viruses, 4
  reported AIDS cases, 114
  social dimensions of AIDS, 113
Honduras
  AIDS cases, 59
Hong Kong
  AIDS epidemiology, 55
Horwitz, Jerome P., 92
Hospitals
  AIDS patient expenses, 110
  care of AIDS patients, 115–116
Host cells
  HIV infection, 89
  HIV therapies, 94, 95
Host-cell proteins, 87
HTLV's (see human T-lymphotropic virus)
Huberman, Joel A., 87
Human B-cell lymphotropic virus (HBLV), 9
Human herpes virus 6 (HHV-6), 9–10
Human immunodeficiency virus (HIV), 1, 3, 4–11, 112
  blocking infection, 83
  cellular aspects, 75–84
  clinical course of, 63–73
  discovery of, 1
  envelope protein, 101
  epidemiology in U.S., 39–49
  genetic structure, 18
  infection steps, 107
  international epidemiology, 51–61
  life cycle, 87–89
  molecular biology of, 13–25
  origins of, 27–37

  replication, 87–89
  similarity to SIV, 30
  spread in and from Africa, 9
  spread of, 10
  test for, 42
  therapies, 10, 85–99
  transmission of, 52, 63, 64, 112
  vaccines, 101–110
  (See also acquired immune deficiency syndrome)
Human immunodeficiency virus 1 (HIV-1), 7, 9, 109
  genetic organization, 36
  international epidemiology, 52
  proteins, 31
  West Africa, 34–37, 53
Human immunodeficiency virus 2 (HIV-2), 7–9
  genetic organization, 36
  international epidemiology, 52
  macaque monkeys, 108–109
  rate of African infection, 35
  West Africa, 34–37, 53
Human T-lymphotropic virus type I (HTLV-I), 2, 3–4, 28
  genetic structure, 17, 19
Human T-lymphotropic virus type II (HTLV-II), 2, 3, 28
  genetic structure, 17, 19
Human T-lymphotropic virus type III (HTLV-III), 4
Human T-lymphotropic virus type IV (HTLV-IV), 34
Human T-lymphotropic viruses (HTLV's), 3, 4
  leukemia, 37
Humoral response to infection, 102, 105
Hybridization
  HIV therapies, 95
Hyperactivity
  B cells and HIV infection, 67, 70
Hypervariable loop, 24

Illinois
  premarital screening for AIDS, 115
Immune-stimulation complexes, 108
Immune system
  AIDS research, 120–121
  breakdown in AIDS victims, 2
  cell death, 22
  herpes virus infection, 9–10
  HIV infection, 9–10, 11, 64–68, 69, 70, 72, 75, 80, 89, 101, 105–106
  HIV therapies, 90, 96, 97
  HIV vaccines, 102

  retroviruses, 103
Immunoglobulin molecule
  HIV therapies, 90–91
Imperial Cancer Research Fund, 108
Industrialized countries
  AIDS patterns, 52
Infants
  HIV infection, 46
Insect vectors
  transmission of HIV, 46–47
Insurance
  AIDS patient costs, 119–120
  care of AIDS patients, 116
Insurance companies
  AIDS education programs, 118
Intelligence quotient (IQ)
  AIDS therapies, 97
Interferons
  HIV therapies, 88, 96
  immune system, 23
  (See also alpha-interferons)
Interleukin-1
  immune system, 23
Intestines
  HIV infection, 13
Intravenous drug abusers (see drug users, intravenous)
Israel
  AIDS cases, 59
Italy
  AIDS epidemiology, 57, 59
Ito, Masahiko, 91
Ivory Coast
  HIV infection, 37

Jamaica
  AIDS cases, 59
Japan
  AIDS epidemiology, 55, 59
  AIDS vaccines, 110
  HTLV origins, 28
Japanese macaque monkey
  STLV, 28
Javaherian, Kashi, 106
Jenner, Edward, 102
Johns, David G., 97
Johnson, Robert Wood, Foundation, 118
Judgment
  and HIV infection, 69

Kaiser Family Foundation, 115
Kaiser-Permanente Medical Group, 119
Kanki, Phyllis J., 9
Kaposi's sarcoma, 40, 64, 70
  therapies, 85
Karon, John, 48
Kennedy, Ronald C., 84, 89, 108
Kinases
  HIV therapies, 92
Kinshasa, Zaire
  AIDS cases, 54
  economic losses from AIDS, 120

Klatzmann, David, 3, 6, 76
Koop, C. Everett, 101
Kuno, Sachiko, 91
Kyotera, Uganda
  AIDS cases, 51

Landau, Ned, 82
Larder, Brendan A., 92
Larson, S. M., 87
Lasky, Larry, 82
Latency period
  between HIV infection
    and AIDS, 41, 48, 58,
    106, 110, 112
Latin America
  AIDS epidemiology, 52,
    57, 58
  blood screening, 60
LAV (see
  lymphadenopathy-
  associated virus)
Legionella
  and AIDS, 68–69
Leibowitch, Jacques, 2
Letvin, Norman L., 30
Leu3a
  HIV infection, 80–84
Leukemias
  childhood, 99
  hairy-cell, 2
  HTLV, 37
  mice, 103
  regulatory genes, 17
  and retroviruses, 2
Levy, Jay A., 77, 79
Liability
  AIDS vaccine testing, 110
Lifson, Jeffrey D., 89
Lipids
  HIV, 87
Liposomes
  AIDS vaccines, 107
Littman, Dan R., 78, 82
Long terminal repeats
  (LTR's), 14
  HIV, 18, 19, 20
  HIV therapies, 95
Los Angeles, California
  AIDS epidemiology, 40
Lymphadenopathy, 3, 40
Lymphadenopathy, chronic
  HIV infection, 40, 65, 67
Lymphadenopathy-
  associated virus (LAV),
  3–4
Lymphocytes
  HIV infection, 7
  simian AIDS, 30
Lymphoid cancer
  HIV-related viruses, 28
Lymphokines, 102, 105
Lymphomas
  causes, 2
  and HIV infection, 70
  therapy, 85

Macaque monkeys
  HIV infection, 108–109
  simian AIDS, 27
  SIV, 7–9
  STLV infection, 28
McClure, Myra O., 77–78
McDougal, J. Steven, 76, 77

Macrophages, 80
  and antibodies, 89
  HIV infection, 6, 7, 13,
    22, 23, 64, 65, 102, 105
Maddon, Paul, 76–77, 78
Male-to-female ratio of
  AIDS cases, 52–53,
  113–114
Mammalian cells, 87
Matsukura, Makoto, 95
Matsushita, Shuzo, 89
M'Boup, Soylemane, 33
Medicaid
  AIDS patient costs, 116,
    119, 120
Medical care
  AIDS patients, 118–120
Medical costs
  AIDS patients, 118–120
Medicine, practice of
  precautions against AIDS,
    115–116
Memory
  and HIV infection, 69
"Memory" cells, 102, *105*
Merck Sharp & Dohme, 103
Merigan, Thomas C., Jr., 97
Messenger RNA (mRNA),
  14, 18–19
  genetic regulation, 17
  HIV infection, 20, 80
  HIV therapies, *88*, 95
  rev protein, 23
  viral growth, *21*
Metropolitan Life Insurance
  Company, 118
Mexico
  AIDS epidemiology, 52, *59*
MicroGeneSys, Inc., 107
Mice
  CD4 receptor and HIV,
    77, 82, 84
  leukemia, 103
Microglial cells, 22
Middle East
  AIDS epidemiology, 53
Military service applicants
  HIV infection rate, 48–49
Minority communities
  AIDS cases, 114, 115
  public-health measures,
    120
Mitsuya, Hiroaki, 87, 91
Miyoshi, Isao, 28
Molluscum contagiosum
  and HIV infection, 70
Monkeys
  HIV infection, 82,
    108–109
  HIV-related viruses, 27–32
  simian AIDS, 27
  SIV infection, 7–9, 34
  STLV infection, 28
Monoclonal antibodies, *90*
  HIV infection, 76, 80–84
  HIV therapies, 89
Monocytes
  HIV infection, 13, 22, 23,
    64, 65
Montagnier, Luc, 2–3, 4, 7,
  9, 14, 35
Morbidity rate
  U.S. AIDS cases, 39

Morehouse College School
  of Medicine, 115
Morein, Bror, 108
Morgan, W. Meade, 48
Mortality rate
  AIDS cases, 39, 54, 58
Moss, Bernard, 108
Mothers
  and transmission of HIV
    to children, 2, 10, 43,
    46, 52
mRNA (see messenger RNA)
Mucous membrane
  infections
  and HIV, 68
Mutations
  CD4 gene, 82
  cell replication, 24
  HIV, 24, 89, 103–105
  HIV therapies, 92
Mycobacterial diseases, 69
Myxoma
  in rabbits, 32, 33

Nabel, Gary J., 95
Nairobi, Kenya
  AIDS cases, 54
Names Project AIDS quilt,
  112
National AIDS Awareness
  Test, 113, 118
National Cancer Institute
  (NCI)
  HIV therapies, 97
National Cooperative
  Vaccine Development
  Groups, 110
National Institute of Allergy
  and Infectious Diseases,
  107
National Institutes of
  Health (NIH)
  AIDS expenditures, 116
  HIV therapies, 96
nef gene, 19, *20*, 24
nef protein, 20–21, 23
Negative-regulatory element
  sequence (NRE)
  HIV, 19
  nef protein, *21*, 24
Nervous system (see central
  nervous system)
Netherlands
  AIDS cases, *59*
Neurological disorders
  and HIV infection, 69
Neuropathy, peripheral
  HIV therapies, 97
Newborns
  HIV-infected, 119
New England Regional
  Primate Research
  Center, 28, 30, 109
New York City
  AIDS and tuberculosis, 119
  AIDS cases, 114
  AIDS expenditures, 117
  AIDS memorial quilt, *112*
  HIV-infected women
    giving birth, 119

medical care costs for
  AIDS patients, 120
New York City Department
  of Health
  AIDS education program,
    118
New York State
  AIDS epidemiology, 40,
    56, 114
  AIDS expenditures, 117
New York Life Insurance
  Company, 118
New Zealand
  AIDS epidemiology, 52,
    53, 55, *59*
NF-κB, 20, 95
Nilsson, Lennart, *1*
North Africa
  AIDS epidemiology, 52, 53
North America
  AIDS epidemiology, 53
Norway
  AIDS cases, 59
NRE (see negative-
  regulatory element
  sequence)
Nucleoside analogues
  HIV therapies, 92–94
Nucleoside triphosphates, 92
Nucleotides
  cell killing, 24
  genetic regulation, 17
  HIV, 13–14
  HIV and SIV, 30, 34
  HIV therapies, 94–95
Nursery facilities
  HIV-infected newborns,
    119
Nurses
  care of AIDS patients, 116

Oceania
  AIDS epidemiology, 55
OKT4a
  HIV infection, 80, 82
Old World primates
  HTLV infection, 28
  STLV infection, 28
Oligodeoxynucleotides
  HIV therapies, 98
Oligonucleotides
  HIV therapies, *88*, 94–95
Oncogen, 108
Opportunistic-defined
  AIDS, 68
Opportunistic infections
  and AIDS, 67
  and helper *T* cells, 89
  and HIV, 63, 68, 69
  therapy, 85
Oral hairy leukemia, 68, *69*
Ostertag, Wolfram, 87
Özel, Muhsin, *9*, *11*

p17, 108
p25 (or p24), 4, *31*
p55, *31*
Pacific
  AIDS epidemiology, 53,
    55–56
Palker, Thomas J., 106
Patas monkeys
  SIV infection, 30

Pediatrics (*see* children)
Pentamidine (pentamidine isethionate), 40, 69
People With AIDS Coalition, *117*
Perinatal transmission of AIDS, 45, 46, 114
  international epidemiology, 52, 53
  prevention of, 60
Peripheral-blood lymphocytes
  HIV infection, 76
Peripheral-blood monocytes, 80
Perno, Carlo-Federico, 97
Peterson, Andrew, 82
Philippines
  prostitutes and HIV, 55
Phosphonoformate, *98*
Phosphorothioate oligodeoxynucleotides, *98*
Phosphorothioates, antisense, 95
Phosphorylation, 92
Pizzo, Philip A., 97
Pneumocystis carinii pneumonia (PCP), 40, 41, 63, 68, 69, 96
pol gene, *18*, 36
Polio vaccines, 103
Polymerase
  RNA, 20
  viral genetic information, 14
Popovic, Mikulas, 6, 76
Population groups
  U.S. AIDS cases, *44*
Portland, Oregon
  AIDS prevention program, 114
Portugal
  AIDS cases, *59*
Pre-AIDS, 4
Pregnancy
  prevention of AIDS, 60
Premarital screening for HIV, 115
Prevention of AIDS, 114–115
  education program, 60
Primates
  HIV infection, 82
  HIV-related viruses, 27–32
  retroviruses, *28*
  SIV, 7–9, 30–32
  STLV infection, 28
Prostitutes
  African AIDS epidemiology, 53–54
  HIV infection, 35, 55–56
  SIV-related viruses in Africans, 33–34
Proteases, 9
  HIV infection, 14
  virion assembly, *16*
Protein kinase, 19
Proteins
  cross-reactivity of viruses, *31*
  flow of genetic information, 1

HIV, 14, 15, *16*, 20–21
HIV and SIV, 30
SIV, *31, 34*
viral genetic information, 14, *15*
  (*See also* p17; p25; p55)
Proteins, foreign
  breakdown of immune system, 2
Proteins, host-cell, 87
Proteins, regulatory, 18–19
  viral growth, *21*
Proteins, viral, 87
  HIV infection, 18–19, 28, 64, *66*, 75, 78, 80, 84, 87–89
  HIV therapies, 94–96
  p25, 4
  viral growth, *21*
Provirus, 2, 14, *15*
Pseudotype assay, 76
Public health
  AIDS epidemic, 120
  AIDS programs, 114–115
Public Health Service, U.S.
  AIDS epidemiology, 47
  AIDS expenditures, 116
  AIDS vaccines, 110
  HIV infection estimates, 58
  predicted AIDS cases, 119
Purines, 92
Putney, Scott D., 106
Pyrimidines, 92

Rabbits
  HIV infection, 109
  myxoma, 32, *33*
rCD4, 90
Reagents
  cause of AIDS, *11*
  typing viruses, 4
Receptor-mediated endocytosis, 77–78, *79*
Recombinant DNA methods
  soluble CD4, 90
Redfield, Robert R., 7
Replication
  cell death, 22
  HIV, 13, 15, 17, 64–65, *66*, 72, 76, 87
  HIV and mutations, 24
  HIV therapies, 91, 95, 97
  SIV and HIV genetic organization, 36
  viral growth, 18, 19, 87
Retrovir (AZT), 63
Retroviruses, 1–3
  and cancer, 2, 3
  dormancy and therapy, 85
  genetic information, 14
  genetic regulation, 15–17, 19
  HIV, 4
  HIV-related, 27
  HIV therapies, 92
  mutations and cell replication, 24
  proteins, 30
  primates and, *28*
  treatment of, 10, 87
  vaccines against, 103
  virus-host relation, 32
Reverse transcriptase, 2, *4*, 14

HIV, 87–88
HIV therapies, 91–92, 94
lymphadenopathy, 3
rev gene, 18–19, *20*, 23
rev protein, 21
Ribaviran, *98*
Ribonuclease, 14
Ribosomal-hybridization arrest, 95
Richman, Douglas D., 96
Rifabutin, *98*
Risk factors for AIDS, 39, 54
RNA, viral
  genetic information, 14, *15*
  HIV infection, 3, 4, *16*, *18*, 20, 64, 80, 87–88, 91
  HIV therapies, 94–95, 96
  mutations and cell replication, 24
  retroviruses, 1–2
  (*See also* messenger RNA)
RNase H, 94
Rozenbaum, Willy, 3
Rusche, James R., 106
Rwanda
  AIDS epidemiology, *51*, 53–54

Saatchi & Saatchi Compton, Inc., 118
Sahel region
  AIDS epidemiology, 53
SAIDS (*see* simian AIDS)
Saliva
  risk of HIV infection, 46
Salk, Jonas, 108
Salmonella
  and AIDS, 69
San Francisco, California
  AIDS cases, 114
  AIDS medical care costs, 120
Sattentau, Quentin J., 80–82, 84
Scandinavia
  AIDS epidemiology, 53
Schäfer, Werner, 103
Schooley, Robert T., 96
Seed, Brian, 82
Senegal
  SIV-related viruses, 33
Septra/Bactrium, 69
Serological studies
  AIDS cases, 42
Sexual behavior
  homosexual men and AIDS, 48
  in sub-Saharan Africa and AIDS, 54
Sexual intercourse
  spread of viruses, 2
  transmission of HIV, 10, 43–45, 52
  U.S. epidemiology of AIDS, 40, 41
Sexually transmitted diseases
  risk of HIV infection, 54
Shanti Project, 117
Shaw, George M., 6
Shearer, Gene M., 96
Simian AIDS (SAIDS), 30 *31, 32*

Simian immunodeficiency virus (SIV), 7–9, 27, *28*
  antibodies, 81
  genetic organization, 36
  and HIV proteins, 30
  hosts, 30–33
  related viruses in Africa, 33–34
  similarity to HIV, 30
  vaccines, 109
Simian *T*-lymphotropic virus (STLV), 28
Singapore
  AIDS epidemiology
  SIV macaque monkey, 7–9
Skin infections
  and HIV, 68
Slim Disease, 60, 80
Smallpox vaccine, 102
Smith Kline & French Laboratories, 90
Social dimensions of AIDS, 111–121
Sodroski, Joseph G., 96
Sontag, Susan, 111
South America
  AIDS epidemiology, *53, 59*
Spain
  AIDS epidemiology, 57
Sperm
  breakdown of immune system, 2
Stein, Barry S., 77–78
STLV (*see* simian *T*-lymphotropic virus)
Sub-Saharan Africa
  AIDS epidemiology, 54
Sugar molecules
  HIV envelope protein, *101*, 106
Sweden
  AIDS epidemiology, 57, *59*
  AIDS vaccines, 110
Switzerland
  AIDS cases, *59*
Swollen glands (*see* lymphadenopathy)
Syncytia, 9
  cell death, 22
  HIV infection, 65, *66*, 76, 77, 78, 89
  HIV therapies, 91, 96
Syphilis
  decline of, 48
  and HIV infection, 45, 54

T cells, 76
  AIDS vaccines, 108
  and AZT, 92
  cell death, 22
  HIV infection, 10, 13, 20, 80
  HTLV-I, 2
  immortality, 28
  immune response to infection, *105*
T cells, helper (*T*4 lymphocytes), 64–69, 72, 102
  depletion in AIDS patients, 2
  HIV infection, 6–7, 9, 10, 13, 17, 22, 75, 76, 80, *88*, 102

HIV therapies, 89, 90, 96, 97
immune response to infection, *105*
lymphadenopathy-associated virus, 3
SIV, 30
T cells, killer (*T*8 lymphocytes), 3, 22, 64, 76, 102
Tanzania
AIDS epidemiology, *51*, 53
TAR sequence (*see trans*-acting responsive sequence)
tat gene, 4, 17, 18–19, *20*, 23
Taylor, Elizabeth, 117
T-cell leukemias, 2
Temin, Howard M., 2
Thailand
AIDS epidemiology, 56
Therapeutic index of drugs, 87
Therapies, AIDS, 85–99, 119
Thrush, 68, *69*
Thymidine, 92
Thymidine triphosphate, 92
Thymine, *93*
Thymus gland
HIV infection, 22
Tissue-dendritic cells
HIV infection, 65
Tissues, body
HIV infection, *81*
Toxicity
HIV therapies, 97–99
Toxoplasmosis
and AIDS, 68
trans-acting responsive sequence (TAR sequence), 17
Translation arrest
HIV therapies, 95

Treatment centers for AIDS, 114, 119
Trimming glycosidases, 96
Triphosphates, 92
Tuberculosis
and HIV infection, 35–36, 68, 119

Ueno, Ryuji, 91
Uganda
AIDS education programs, *60*
AIDS epidemiology, *51*, 53, 58
United Kingdom
AIDS epidemiology, 57, *59*
United States
AIDS epidemic, 113–114
AIDS epidemiology, 39–49, 52, 59
AIDS expenditures, 116–117
AIDS patient costs, 118–120
AIDS public-health measures, 114–115
blood tests for AIDS, 11
children with AIDS, 119
geographical distribution of AIDS, 114
HIV infection estimates, 30, 58
practice of medicine and AIDS, 115–116
SIV-related viruses, 33–34
transmission of AIDS, 114
U.S. Presidential Commission on the HIV Epidemic, 114, 120
University College London, 108
Urban areas
African AIDS cases, *51*, 54

Vaccines
AIDS, 10, 101–110, 120–121
anti-CD4 monoclonal antibodies, 84
Venereal disease
risk of HIV infection, 45
Vesicular stomatitis virus (VSV), 76
vif gene, 21–22
Viral binding
inhibiting, 89–91
Viral integrase, 94
Viral proteins (*see* proteins, viral)
Viral Technologies, Inc., 108
Viruses
cell infection, 87
and HIV infection, 14–15, *16*
structure, *4*
treatment of, 10
Volunteers
AIDS vaccines, 110
vpr gene, 20
vpu gene, 20, 30, 37
vpx gene, 30, 37
VSV (*see* vesicular stomatitis virus)
VSV (HIV) pseudotypes, 76

Walter Reed Army Medical Center, 64
Walter Reed classification system of HIV, 64, 65–69, 70–71
Warwick, Dionne, 115
Weiss, Robin A., 6
Wellcome Research Laboratories, *87*, 96
West Africa
AIDS epidemiology, 7, 53

HIV infection, 52
HIV-2, 34–37
SIV-related viruses, 33–34
West Germany
AIDS cases, *59*
Western Europe
AIDS epidemiology, 52, 53, 56–57
Women
AIDS cases, 114
HIV infection in Africa, 54
Wong-Staal, Flossie, 4, 6, 106
World AIDS Foundation, 11
World Health Assembly, 52, 120
World Health Organization (WHO), 11
Global Program on AIDS, 51, 120
reported AIDS cases, *55*, 58, 59–61
World Summit of Ministers of Health, 120

Yugoslavia
AIDS cases, *59*

Zagury, Daniel, 108
Zaire
AIDS epidemiology, *51*, 53–54, 58, 59
AIDS vaccines, 108
economic losses from AIDS, 120
Zambia
AIDS epidemiology, *51*, 53, 59, 120
Zamecnik, Paul C., 94
Zavada, Jan, 76
Zidovudine (*see* azidothymidine)
Zon, Gerald, 95